MAJOR TOPICS IN TYPE 1 DIABETES

Edited by **Kenia Pedrosa Nunes**

Major Topics in Type 1 Diabetes
http://dx.doi.org/10.5772/59335
Edited by Kenia Pedrosa Nunes

Contributors

Laura Nabors, Denise Faustman, Miriam Davis, Ippei Watari, Katarzyna A. Podyma-Inoue, Mona Abbassy, Takashi Ono, Yoel Greenwald, M.Graça Pereira, Ana Cristina Almeida, Engrácia Leandro, Shereen Abdelghaffar, Michal Cohen, Naim Shehadeh, Nehama Zukerman-Levin, Smadar Shilo, Kenia Pedrosa Nunes

Published by InTech

Janeza Trdine 9, 51000 Rijeka, Croatia

Publishing Process Manager Iva Lipovic

Technical Editor InTech DTP team

Cover InTech Design team

First published November, 2015

Printed in Croatia

Additional hard copies can be obtained from orders@intechopen.com

Major Topics in Type 1 Diabetes, Edited by Kenia Pedrosa Nunes

p. cm.

ISBN 978-953-51-2204-3

For EU product safety concerns:
IN TECH d.o.o., Prolaz Marije Krucifikse Kozulić 3, 51000 Rijeka, Croatia,
info@intechopen.com or visit our website at intechopen.com.

Meet the editor

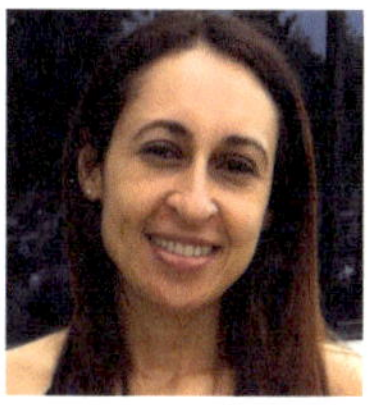

Dr. Kenia Pedrosa Nunes is a vascular biologist who studies diseases such as diabetes, hypertension, and especially erectile dysfunction (ED). She received her master's degree in Molecular and Biochemistry Pharmacology and her Ph.D. in Physiology from the Federal University of Minas Gerais, Brazil. As a postdoctoral fellow at the Medical College of Georgia, Dr. Nunes specialized in vascular function and dysfunction and started to study how the immune system contributes to the development of hypertension and diabetes-associated ED. The role of the immune system in diabetes and cardiovascular disease is now being investigated by many scientists around the world. Dr. Nunes's research has been supported by the American Heart Association (AHA) since 2009. She is a professor of Human Physiology and Anatomy at the Florida Institute of Technology, where she continues to work on rewarding projects involving diabetes and hypertension, using animal models to investigate different pathways leading to vascular diseases and new treatment targets. She has to her credit more than 20 peer-reviewed manuscripts, 6 book chapters, and an international patent regarding pharmaceutical compositions to improve vasculogenic erectile function.

Contents

Preface

According to the World Health Organization, diabetes will be the seventh leading cause of death in 2030. Diabetes is a disease that affects the whole family, especially when a child is diagnosed. Type 1 diabetes (T1D) is one of the most common endocrine disorders of children, and the incidence of diabetes is steadily increasing. T1D is largely considered an autoimmune disorder resulting from the specific destruction of the pancreatic beta-cells that produce insulin. However, T1D pathophysiology is still not completely understood, and although insulin and other therapies ameliorate the manifestations of the disease, no cure is currently available.

The existing scientific books on diabetes offer vast amounts of information regarding the disease. This book focuses on lesser explored topics regarding T1D, subjects that are important from the point of view of future treatments of diabetes. While the book focuses on a few issues in the broad area of T1D, these topics have been discussed by the scientific community as being very relevant and in need of further research in order to significantly increase our knowledge and management of T1D. It is a book that calls upon experts from around the world who communicate the most accurate scientific information in a way that will be useful for medical students as well as diabetic patients and their families.

I wish to express gratitude to all who have helped in the compilation of this small but substantial book. In addition, I want to thank the readers on behalf of all the authors who contributed to this book. I hope this work will add to the continuing debate over how to better handle diabetic complications and provide an overview about current possibilities to forestall them, in addition to highlighting new insights into T1D. Suggestions and feedback would be most welcome.

Kenia Pedrosa Nunes
Department of Biological Sciences,
Florida Institute of Technology,
Melbourne, FL, USA

Chapter 1

The Innate Immune System via Toll-Like Receptors (TLRs) in Type 1 Diabetes - Mechanistic Insights

Kenia Pedrosa Nunes, Eric Guisbert, Theodora Szasz and Clinton Webb

Additional information is available at the end of the chapter

http://dx.doi.org/10.5772/61925

Abstract

Type 1 diabetes (T1D) is a form of diabetes mellitus resulting from the lack of insulin secretion by the pancreatic beta cells and which accounts for approximately 5% of the total number of patients with diabetes worldwide. T1D is one of the most common endocrine disorders of children, and its incidence is steadily increasing. T1D is largely considered an autoimmune disorder resulting from the specific destruction of the pancreatic beta-cells that produce insulin. However, T1D pathophysiology is still not completely understood, and although insulin and other therapies ameliorate the manifestations of the disease, no cure is currently available. Traditionally, T1D has been thought of as a condition of cellular adaptive immunity, but evidence exists that components of the innate immune system, such as Toll-like receptors (TLRs), play a critical role in T1D development. TLRs have a central role in sensing microbial infections as well as endogenous alarm signals and trigger the release of inflammatory cytokines. The involvement of these receptors in the pathophysiology of several chronic diseases has become a major research interest, and in the last two decades, many studies have suggested the involvement of the innate immune system in the mechanism triggering T1D. Furthermore, microvascular complications in diabetic patients result in considerable morbidity, particularly diabetic nephropathy, retinopathy, and atherosclerosis. A hallmark of diabetic vascular pathology is inflammation and endothelial dysfunction. Recent literature suggests that TLR signaling is involved in vascular inflammation and endothelial dysfunction and that TLR activation may play a crucial role in diabetic microangiopathy. However, the mechanisms by which TLRs and their ligands contribute to T1D are not yet clear, and further investigation is needed. The goal of the present chapter is to address the contribution of TLRs to the mechanisms leading to the development and progression of T1D and to review current possibilities of targeting TLRs to forestall diabetic complications.

Keywords: Toll-like receptors, type 1 diabetes, DAMPS, innate immune system, microangiopathy

1. Introduction

The innate immune system is the first line of defense against invading organisms and other dangerous events in our body. Unlike the acquired immune system, innate immunity identifies the presence of harm via pattern recognition receptors (PRRs). Toll-like receptors (TLRs) are one of the most important classes of PRRs for sensing harmful signals. TLRs can recognize two types of molecules: (1) conserved pathogen molecules such as lipopolysaccharide (LPS), proteins, and nucleic acids expressed by microbes, viruses, bacteria, and fungi, which are known as pathogen-associated molecular patterns or PAMPS [1-2] and (2) endogenous molecules released from damaged cells or tissues such as HMGB-1, HSP60, and C-reactive protein called damage-associated patterns or DAMPS [3]. To date, ten TLRs have been identified in humans (TLR1–TLR10) and twelve in mice (TLR1–TLR9 and TLR11–TLR13). Most TLRs are located on the cell surface, except for TLR3, TLR7, TLR8, and TLR9, which are expressed in the intracellular compartment, the endosome [4].

All TLRs share their intracellular domain with the interleukin-1-receptor (IL-1R) family. Two major intracellular signaling pathways are triggered by TLRs, one that is canonical and dependent on myeloid differentiation primary response protein 88 (MyD88) and another that is noncanonical and MyD88-independent (Figure 1) pathway. MyD88 binds to TLRs upon activation and is essential for the induction of inflammatory cytokines via TLRs. All TLRs, except TLR3, can activate a MyD88-dependent pathway, which involves mitogen-activated kinases and leads to the transcription of pro-inflammatory genes through the activation of nuclear factor κB (NF-κB). TLR3 activates the TRIF-mediated pathway, a MyD88-independent pathway that in turn activates interferon regulatory factor 3 (IRF-3), inducing the expression of interferons (IFNs) [5]. TLR pathway activation results in the activation of the inhibitor of NF-κB kinase (IKK) complex and the transcription factor nuclear factor κB (NF-κB). NF-κB has been extensively studied as a regulator of inflammatory mediators, including tumor necrosis factor alpha (TNF-α). Increased levels of interleukin 1 beta (IL-1β) and TNF-α have been correlated with an expression of TLR2 and TLR4 on monocytes from T1D patients [6] (Figure 1).

Type 1 diabetes (T1D) is a disease in which the pancreatic insulin-producing beta-cells are lost or destroyed, usually via autoimmune mechanisms. Consequently, slow and progressive islet beta-cell impairment and total loss of insulin secretion are observed [7-8]. How the disease is triggered is unknown; however, research in animal models of T1D supports the hypothesis that microbial infection and/or innate immune system activation play an important role in disease mechanisms [9]. Several lines of evidence suggest that T1D progression is strongly heritable [10-11]. However, in addition to genetic factors, environmental factors such as chemicals, infections, and components of early childhood diet might contribute to T1D onset [12]. The development of T1D can be classified into two stages. In the first stage, called insulitis, Langerhans islets in the pancreas are progressively infiltrated by cells of the immune system, especially T cells and macrophages (Figure 2). In the second stage, most beta-cells are destroyed by the infiltrating immune cells. Apoptosis of pancreatic beta-cells is the last step in the initial pathogenesis of T1D [13]. Regardless of the progress toward the last step of T1D development,

http://dx.doi.org/10.5772/61925

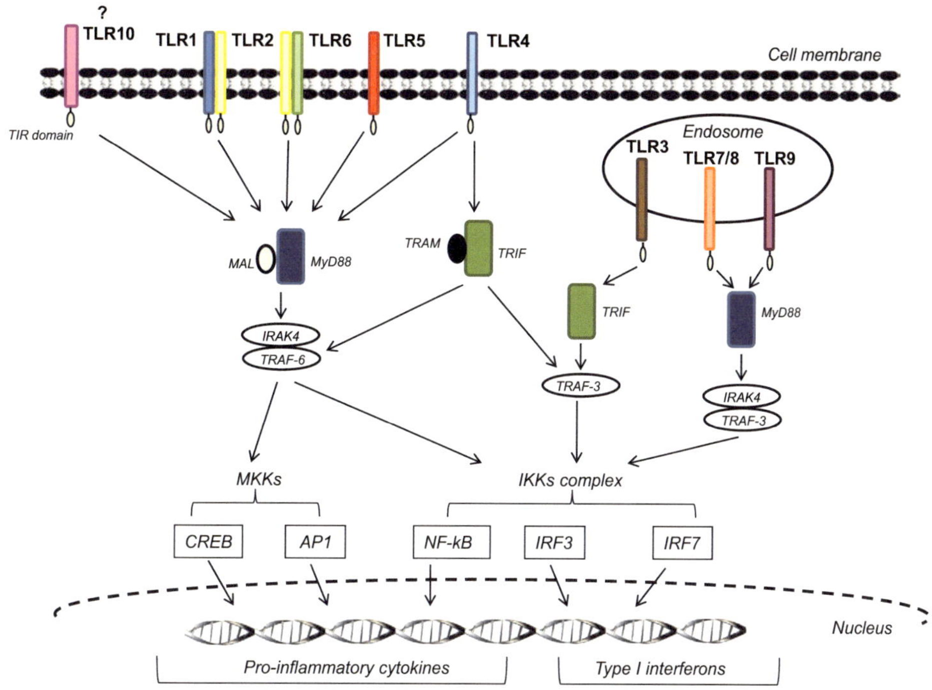

Figure 1. Ten human TLRs and their pathways. Signaling pathways activated by TLRs might be MyD88 dependent or independent. MyD88 is an adaptor molecule, which recruits IRAK and induces phosphorylation. IRAK associates with TRAF6 or TRAF3, leading to the activation of IKK complex or MKKs and resulting in the activation of NF-κB and other important transcription factors (CREB and AP1). The activation of a MyD88-dependent pathway leads to induction of inflammatory cytokines or type I interferons (IFNs). All TLRs, except TLR3, can activate MyD88. The MyD88-independent pathway is called TRIF-mediated pathway (TIR-domain-containing adaptor inducing an NF-κB). TLR4 can also utilize the TRIF-related adaptor molecule (TRAM) for the activation of NF-κB. In order to switch signaling from MyD88 to TRIF, TLR4 moves from plasma membrane to the endosomes. Little is known about TLR10 and its ligands, but this receptor may heterodimerize with TLR1 and TLR2. The activation of TLRs especially TLR2 and TLR4 pathways leads to complications that are associated with the pathogenesis of diabetes. CRBE: cyclic AMP-responsive element binding-protein; AP1: activator protein 1.

the initial step, triggering anti-islet autoimmunity, is still unclear and this is one of the most relevant issues in the field of autoimmune diseases.

Generally, TLR-expressing innate immune cells trigger the initial actions against dangerous signals, which later lead to the activation of T and B cells of the adaptive immune system. Although the primary function of TLRs is linked to the innate immunity, there are no reasons why TLRs may not have a direct function on adaptive immunity, and it has been recently demonstrated that TLRs are also expressed not only in cells from the innate immune but also in T and B cells [14-16]. Continuous release of DAMPs from damaged cells and tissues may maintain the activation of the innate immune system in diseases with long-term low-level inflammation. Therefore, the participation of innate immunity via TLRs not only in acute but also in chronic disease has been recently speculated in the literature. The expression of TLRs in T or B cells has been suggested to provide a cell intrinsic mechanism for innate signals

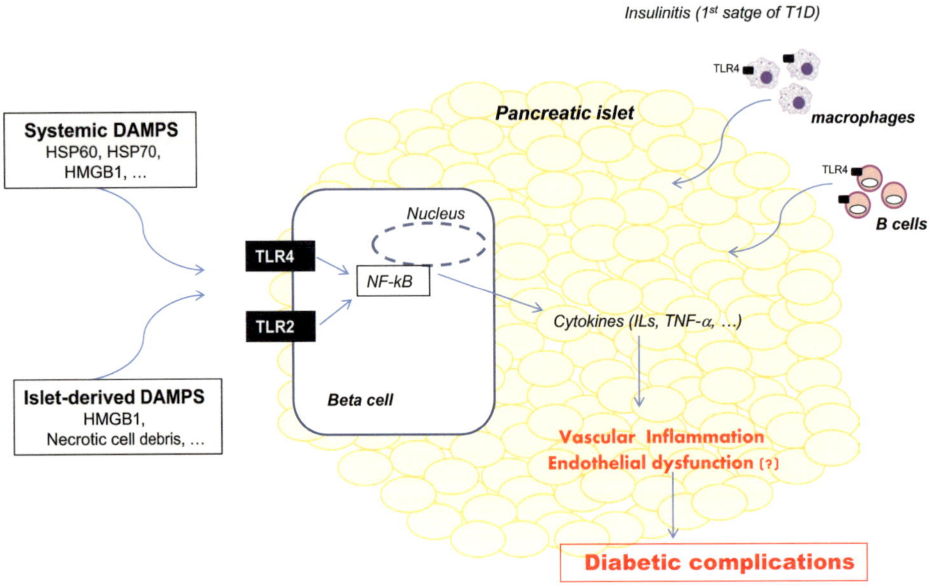

Figure 2. Involvement of TLR2 and TLR4 in the development of T1D. TLR2 and TLR4 on islet beta-cells senses expression changes in DAMPS such as HMGB1 and contribute to the initiation of T1D. Activation of TLR2 and TLR4 leads to NF-κB activation and pro-inflammatory cytokines production, which play a part in T1D inflammatory process and possibly endothelial dysfunction resulting in diabetic vascular complications. In addition, in T1D, the pancreas is progressively infiltrated by cells of the immune system such as macrophages and B-cells which express TLR2 and TLR4.

regulating adaptive immune responses [3, 16], which suggest the TLR-mediated activation of innate immunity may be controlling chronic disorders. However, the exact role of the innate immunity and TLRs in chronic diseases such as T1D is still under discussion.

TLRs play a major role in the development of several pancreatic diseases [17]. In the last decade, the involvement of the innate immune system in diabetes development and complications has been highlighted and investigated by many authors [18-19]. The idea that the initial event in the pathogenesis of autoimmune T1D comprises sensing of molecular patterns from apoptotic beta cells by TLRs has been suggested in recent papers [8, 20]. In T1D, necrotic beta-cells might stimulate dendritic cells (DCs), which are essential in defending against microbial infections and are involved in initiating and regulating immune responses linked to inflammation [21]. In addition, during the development of T1D, multiple interactions occur between DCs, macrophages, natural killer cells (NKs), and lymphocytes. Ultimately, the activation of these cells leads to induction of inflammatory genes [22]. A proinflammatory state is characteristic of T1D and is manifested by elevated circulating and cellular biomarkers such as augmented plasma levels of C-reactive proteins (CRP), cytokines (IL-1B, TNF, and IL-6), soluble cell protein adhesion, chemokines, etc. These increases are further accentuated in T1D patients with vascular complications [23-24].

Of the various TLRs, TLR2 and TLR4 have an important role in inflammation associated with diabetes. In addition, T1D harbors a considerably elevated risk for progressive atherosclerotic events and TLRs may be involved, but the mechanistic basis for this phenomenon is not completely clear. Likewise, TLRs are involved in the pathogenesis of diabetic microvascular alterations [25]. However, the TLR activation in this diabetic condition and its association with vascular or endothelial dysfunction has not been well characterized. Experimental studies have shown that TLR2 and TLR4 could be important participants in the progression of atherosclerosis in diabetes [6, 26-27]. On the other hand, TLR3, TLR7, and TLR9 seem to be involved in the initiation of TD1 [5, 28].

In this chapter, based on the recent advances in understanding the role of the innate immune system in chronic disease, we focus on the contribution of TLRs to the mechanisms that trigger T1D onset and the development of its complications. This information might provide new insights into possibilities for therapeutic intervention by targeting and modulating the immune system to abrogate or prevent T1D.

2. Contribution of TLRs in the pathogenesis of T1D

Recently, it has become evident that the dysregulation of the innate immune system can precipitate autoimmune diseases, including T1D. Given its essential role in orchestrating innate immune responses, the TLRs may be expected to play a significant role in the T1D development, progression, and its complications. The connections among inflammation, hyperglycemia, and diabetes have clear implications for the immune system. In addition, TLRs activate two types of downstream signaling pathways that lead to the activation of NF-κB with concomitant increase in inflammatory cytokine secretion (Figure 1). Both pathways contribute significantly to the pathophysiology of inflammation in endothelial dysfunction and are relevant to diabetic microangiopathy. Therefore, the key point regarding the involvement of TLRs in T1D and its complications seems to be the inflammatory process.

2.1. TLR2 and TLR4

The activation of the innate immune system via TLRs, in particular, TLR2 and TLR4, seems to play an important role in the development of T1D. Many authors proposed the sensing of DAMPs released from damaged pancreatic β-cells by TLR2 to be first event in the development of T1D [29-30]. The Increased expression of TLR2 and TLR4 in monocytes was described in patients with T1D compared to healthy patients [6]. In addition, the expression of TLR2 is augmented in T1D in both rat and human kidneys and has been associated with vascular complications [31]. Furthermore, T1D patients with microvascular complications showed increases in TLR2 and TLR4 activity in monocytes compared with matched controls [25]. The higher expression of TLR2 and TLR4 is associated with poor glycemic control, while the knockdown of both TLR2 and TLR4 resulted in a 76% decrease in a high glucose-induced NF-κB response, suggesting an additive effect [32-33]. Also, it has been demonstrated that deletion of TLR2 in mice significantly abrogates the proinflammatory state of T1D for up to 14 weeks in mice and improves the wound healing process, supporting a role for TLR2 in promoting inflammation in diabetes [30, 34].

There are ample data supporting an important role for inflammation associated with atherosclerosis in T1D and TLRs may be mediating this process. A recent study demonstrated that TLR2 and TLR4 mediate inflammatory pathways in endothelial cells exposed to high glucose [35], although the precise mechanism by which glucose fluctuations mediate inflammation in endothelial dysfunction is unknown. In apolipoprotein $E^{-/-}$ mice, the deficiency of IP-10 (interferon-gamma-inducible-protein 10) or its receptor (CXCR3) reduces vascular lesion formation. Also, elevated serum IP-10 levels have been shown in diabetes as well as increased monocytic IP-10 in T1D patients, but it is unclear if the patients had complications [36]. TLR4 agonists such as LPS have been shown to induce IP-10 production, and it has been demonstrated that down-regulation of TLR2 and TLR4 abrogates high glucose-induced IP-10 release via NF-κB inhibition [32].

Although many studies have highlighted the involvement of TLRs in the pathogenesis of T1D, TLRs might also have a beneficial role against T1D. Since the cause of T1D and the mechanisms involving this condition are not completely elucidated, the contradiction about the role of the TLRs in T1D could be dependent on the disease stage or how the disease was triggered. T cells, especially CD4 and CD25 T cells, play an important role in the prevention of autoimmunity. These cells not only express different TLRs, including TLR2, but are also functionally regulated directly or indirectly through TLR signaling [37-38]. Recently, it was showed that treatment of prediabetic mice with a synthetic TLR2 agonist diminished T1D and increased the number and function of CD4 and CD25 T cells, also conferring DCs with tolerogenic properties, suggesting that TLR2 signaling improves immunoregulation to prevent T1D [39]. On the other hand, another study suggested that TLR2 and MyD88 was dispensable for development of T1D in non obese diabetic (NOD) mice [40], which exhibit a susceptibility to spontaneous development of autoimmune insulin-dependent diabetes mellitus. NOD mice are a well established model of autoimmune diseases, including human T1D [41]. These data contrast with other reports showing the involvement of TLR2 in the initiation of autoimmune responses directed against beta-cells [42].

In NOD mice, the deletion of TLR4 results in acceleration of diabetes onset and immune cell infiltration of islets [43]. A recent study in the same animal model showed that TLR4 mediates cardiac lipid accumulation and diabetic heart disease [44]. On the contrary, treatment with a TLR4/MD-2 specific agonist monoclonal antibody (UT18) in NOD mice not only prevented T1D but also reversed new T1D onset diagnosed by polyuria, weight loss, and elevated blood glucose [45]. Supporting these results, an agonistic monoclonal antibody to TLR4/MD-2 reverses the development of diabetes in a high percentage of NOD mice. TLR4 antibody treatment increases T regulatory cell numbers in both the periphery and the pancreatic islet, suggesting a novel immunological tool for management of T1D in humans [46]. Taken together, these observations suggest a potential role for TLR2 and TLR4 in the pathology of diabetes. However, the mechanistic details need to be better investigated. Undoubtedly, the majority of existing data suggest that TLRs play a part in T1D, mediating T1D development and its complications, even if it is not clear if this is a beneficial role, a detrimental role, or a combination of the two.

2.2. Other TLRs and T1D

The role of the TLR pathway in the mechanism of T1D has been intensely investigated in the last decade, and it is undeniable that these receptors are involved in the pathogenesis of T1D. However, the majority of the studies are focused on TLR2 and TLR4 and only a few studies have discussed other TLRs such as TLR1, TLR3, TLR7, and TLR9.

To the best of our knowledge, there is only one study showing that TLR1 may be involved in the mechanism of diabetes. In this work, a detailed phenotypic analysis of the diabetes-resistant NOD.C3H-congenic strain 6 was evaluated, and the results suggested that TLR1 pathway is involved in the inflammatory response and the development of T1D controlled by the Idd6 locus [47].

The TLR3 gene codes for an endoplasmic receptor that recognizes dsRNA and plays an important role in the innate immune response initiated by viral infection. Although there are only a few studies reporting a link between T1D and TLR3 gene alterations, polymorphisms in the TLR3 gene seem to be linked to the risk of T1D. In fact, rs5743313 and rs117221827 polymorphisms were associated with an early age at diagnosis and worse glycemic control [48]. However, genotypic data on a small population of South Africans of Zulu origin suggested a weak association of the TLR3 polymorphism C2593T, C2642A, and A2690G with T1D [49]. The hypothesis that viral infections are involved in T1D is based on epidemiological studies [50]. One of the major observations that support a role for a viral etiology of T1D is that in accordance rates for T1D in monozygotic twins are only 50% instead of the expected 100% if the characteristic would be explained only by genetic factors. TLR3 is expressed at high levels in human and mouse pancreatic beta-cells and antigen-presenting DCs, and this receptor activates the TRIF-mediated pathway, which in turn activates interferon regulatory factor (IRF)-3 inducing the expression of IFNs. However, NF-κB may also be activated by TLR3 to upregulate the production of proinflammatory cytokines [5].

TLR7 stimulation activates DCs and T cells to promote autoimmune diabetes in nonobese diabetic (NOD) mice. Treatment with IRS661, an antagonist for TLR7, inhibits the activation of DCs and CD8 T cells, as well as diminishes insulitis and diabetes onset in NOD mice [51]. Daily administration of a specific TLR7 ligand, 1V136, reduces autoimmune disease and modulates DC function [28]. In addition, treatment with 1Z1, an innate immune modulator generated by conjugating a TLR7 ligand to six units of polyethylene glycol (PEG), effectively prevented the clinical onset of hyperglycemia and reduced islet inflammation in NOD mice [52].

The involvement of TLR9 in T1D has been demonstrated in a rat model (diabetes-resistant BioBreeding or BBDR), which developed the disease following virus infection. In this study, disease progression was dependent on TLR9 signaling, leading to the activation of splenic B cells and bone marrow derived DCs [53]. A recent study investigating DCs subpopulations and their responses to TLRs stimulation in T1D patients, and their relatives showed increased TLR9-mediated interferon-alpha production in the first-degree relatives of T1D patients [27].

3. Contribution of TLRs to T1D complications

Diabetes leads to both microvascular and macrovascular complications. Many studies have shown increased levels of inflammatory biomarkers that could predispose to vascular complications. It is undeniable that TLRs are emerging as major factors in many diseases conditions owing to the activation of signaling pathways leading to the expression of inflammatory mediators and induction of immune responses.

Importantly, members of the TLR family play critical roles in the inflammatory components of vascular pathologies, including atherosclerosis [54-55], a condition characterized by inflammation of the vessel wall of the arterial tree. Atherosclerosis is an important vascular complication and the major cause of morbidity and mortality in diabetic patients [56]. Also, diabetes itself is a risk factor for atherosclerosis. Despite the fact that type 1 diabetics are at lower risk for atherosclerotic cardiovascular disease than type 2 diabetics because of the younger age of the former group, the relative risk is 10 times higher in type 1 diabetics than in nondiabetics of similar age [57]. Moreover, T1D has been linked with increased intima media thickness and impaired endothelial function (6), which affects vascular homeostasis leading to complications in diabetes. Lastly, hyperglycemia is a hallmark of diabetes and the role of glucose in the pathogenesis of atherosclerosis has been intensely discussed [58].

Devaraj et al. [30] reported on the role of TLR2 in the proinflammatory state in diabetes and incipient diabetic nephropathy. In TLR2 knockout streptozotocin (STZ)-induced diabetic animals, these authors observed a significant reduction in the NF-κB activity in peritoneal macrophages as well as in the release of various pro-inflammatory cytokines such as IL-6 and IL-8 compared to wild-type diabetic mice. Moreover, TLR2 KO STZ mice showed a significant decreased in albuminuria compared to WT-STZ, as well as increase in podocyte (epithelial cell in the kidneys) number, decrease in podocyte effacement, and a decrease in macrophages in the kidney. This study clearly implicates the TLR pathway in the genesis of a vascular complication in diabetes and demonstrates greater TLR activity in T1D.

Reactive oxygen species (ROS) formed in the vascular wall target a wide range of signaling molecules in both endothelium and vascular smooth muscle and contribute to vascular damage. Vascular dysfunction and remodeling through oxidative damage involves increased production and/or decreased degradation of ROS. One of the main enzymes implicated in vascular ROS generation is NADPH oxidase, although the mechanism behind induction of vascular NADPH oxidase activation in diabetes is less clear [59]. Recently, the role of TLRs in increased ROS levels in diabetes has been investigated [60-61]. It has been shown that the KO of the $P47^{phox}$ subunit of NADPH oxidase prevents diet-induced obesity via upregulation of both TLR2 and TLR4 [61]. A study addressing diabetic retinopathy using human retinal endothelial treated with high glucose showed that hyperglycemia induces TLR2 and TLR4 activation and downstream TLR signaling mediates augmented inflammation possibly via ROS [62], suggesting a mechanism by which TLRs could contribute to vascular damage in diabetes. However, the precise ligands involved in the activation of TLRs by hyperglycemia are still under investigation, and certainly this information will provide new insight for a role of TLRs in diabetes-associated vascular complications.

4. Endogenous ligands (DAMPS) for TLRs in the mechanism of T1D

A large number of endogenous molecules may be potent activators of the innate immune system via TLRs leading to the release of proinflammatory cytokines from monocytes/macrophages. Unfortunately, there are limited data on the levels of endogenous ligands of TLR2 and TLR4 in T1D; however, a significant elevation of some ligands for TLR2 and TLR4 in T2D has been recently found. Overall, S100, fibrinogen, hyaluronan, oxidized LDL, and advanced glycation end products (AGE) showed increased levels in diabetic conditions and may work as DAMPS for TLRs [63]. However, high-mobility group box-1 protein (HMGB1), heat shock proteins (HSPs), and growth arrest-specific 6 protein (GAS6) are the ligands for TLRs specifically associated with T1D have been highlighted in the current literature.

4.1. HMGB1

HMGB1 was initially identified nearly 30 years ago as a chromatin associated protein that is important for transcriptional regulation. HMGB1 helps organize DNA and facilitates the binding of several regulatory protein complexes to DNA [64]. In addition to its role in transcriptional regulation, HMGB1 has been shown to activate proinflammatory responses following its release by necrotic or injured cells into the extracellular environment [65]. This protein may also be actively secreted by monocytes/macrophages. HMGB1 is implicated in the pathogenesis of a number of diseases associated with inflammation and tissue injury [66], and recently, many studies have suggested that HMGB1 acts as an inflammatory trigger in autoimmune diseases working as a DAMP [67]. Although the receptor for advanced glycation end products (RAGE) was the first HMGB1 receptor to be identified, this interaction alone could not justify all of the observed effects of HMGB1 [68]. Many relevant reports have shown that HMGB1 binds not only to RAGE, but also to TLRs [69]. The group of receptors that respond to HMGB1 is still expanding and includes cell membrane expressed TLR4 and TLR2 and endosomal TLR3, TLR7, and TLR9 [70].

To date, the main TLRs implicated in HMGB1 signaling are TLR2 and TLR4, although it is unknown if these receptors are acting independently or together. HMGB1 function is altered in diabetes, and the signaling systems triggered by this protein are not completely understood. The levels of TLRs and HMGB1 have been shown to be increased in patients with T1D [71], and HMGB1 is highly expressed in the cytoplasm of the islets in diabetic mice compared with nondiabetic controls. Furthermore, HMGB1 has been observed to increase in the cytoplasm of the islets during the progression of diabetes [72], and the augmented expression of this protein was observed in the retinas of diabetic patients with retinopathy [73].

HMGB1 polypeptide by itself has a weak proinflammatory activity, but it acquires proinflammatory activity through binding to proinflammatory mediators [74]. It is of interest to note that high glucose concentrations upregulate HMGB1, a ligand to TLR2 and TLR4 known to produce inflammation through NF-κB activation in human endothelial cells [69]. A recent study showed that while infusion of small amounts of glucose results in oxidative and inflammatory stress in patients with T1D, insulin infusion exerts an anti-inflammatory effect by suppression of TLRs and HMGB1 in mononuclear cells of T1D patients [75]. Moreover, it has been suggested that the activation of TLR4 and RAGE by HMGB1 mediates injury and inflammation by the activation of NF-κB in response to hyperglycemia [68]. A study using NOD mice to address the significance of HMGB1 in the natural history of diabetes showed that HMGB1 interacts with TLR4 in isolated islets. By examining the effects of anti-TLR4 antibodies on HMGB1 cell surfacing binding, the authors suggested that TLR4 is the main receptor for HMGB1 on beta-cells and that HMGB1 may signal through TLR4 to selectively impair beta-cells during the progression of T1D [72]. Overall, a considerable body of evidence suggests that a complex set of mechanisms involving HMGB1, RAGE, and TLRs play a significant role in the development of chronic inflammation in diabetes [68].

On the other hand, many studies have shown that HMGB1 has angiogenic properties in promoting endothelial cell sprouting and migration under hypoxic and necrotic conditions [76-77]. There are data suggesting that release of HMGB1 in wounds initiates TLR4-dependent responses that contribute to neovascularization [78]. In addition, research on the transcriptional profiles of angiogenic endothelial cells has revealed HMGB1 as a promising angiogenic factor [79]. Conversely, a potential role for HMGB1 in atherosclerosis [80] is possible, shown by increased HMGB1 expression in atherosclerotic lesions compared with normal arteries. Under some circumstances, HMGB1 may act as a double-edged sword, but it appears that HMGB1 as a ligand for TLRs in T1D plays a detrimental action. Despite these apparent conflicting results, HMGB1 has a central role in mediating local and systemic responses to several stimuli, is involved in TLRs pathways, and may have therapeutic relevance in T1D.

4.2. HSPs

Heat shock proteins (HSPs) were originally identified as a set of proteins that are upregulated by increases in temperature [81]. These proteins were named for their apparent molecular weight, for example, HSP70 and HSP60, and have been shown to be among the most highly conserved proteins in the cell. Some HSPs, like HSP60s, are already abundant proteins that are further upregulated during stressful conditions. Other HSPs, like HSP70, have homologues that are constitutively highly expressed (sometimes referred to as HSC70s) and other homologues that are stress inducible. Most HSPs function as molecular chaperones that assist in the folding of newly synthesized, misfolded, or damaged proteins. Their requirement in protein folding helps to explain the important role of HSPs in both stress and nonstress conditions and the high degree of HSP conservation.

In addition to their primary role in intracellular protein folding, HSPs have been co-opted in a variety of other pathways. HSPs play an important role in cellular pathways involving cellular growth, division, and apoptosis. HSPs have also been implicated in various aspects of immune system modulation [82]. For example, HSPs have been shown to be involved in antigen presentation through their ability to bind and traffic proteins and peptides.

While their primary function is inside the cell, during stress, HSPs can be expressed on cell surfaces or secreted. One of their extracellular functions is the cross presentation of various antigens that they can bind. In addition, extracellular and purified HSP70 and HSP60 have been shown to bind to TLR2 and TLR4, which results in NF-κB activation in a MyD88 and CD14-dependent manner [83]. HSPs can activate immune cells, including B cells, NK cells,

DCs, macrophages, and T cells. However, these results have been somewhat controversial as some HSP preparations have been shown to be contaminated with bacterial molecules, including LPS. Nevertheless, the abundance of HSPs, their high level of conservation, and their roles in cellular stress and inflammation may all help to explain why HSPs have been classified as important components of DAMP signals.

HSP60 and HSP70 have been implicated as key players in T1D. Both mouse models of T1D (NOD mice) and human patients have T cells that recognize and are activated by HSP60 and HSP70 [84-86]. These activated T cells then go to the pancreatic islets and recognize self HSP60 as an autoantigen. Extracellular HSP70 levels are positively correlated with insulin resistance *in vivo* and can cause β-cell dysfunction and death *in vitro* [87]. In mouse models, exogenous HSP60 and immunogenic peptides from HSP60 have been shown to alter the effects of T cells and prevent further β-cell destruction [88]. One peptide, in particular, DiaPep277, has shown promise in phase II clinical trials [89-90]. Phase III clinical trials using this peptide have been completed, but problems with the data analysis have surfaced and a new analysis of the clinical data is currently underway and expected to be completed soon [91-92]. HSP60 and HSP70 have also been implicated in complications of T1D, including atherosclerosis, indicating that they may have multiple roles in T1D [93-95].

4.3. GAS6

Growth arrest-specific 6 (GAS6) protein is another endogenous ligand of TLR2 and TLR4 that has been studied in experimental models of diabetic nephropathy [96], which is the most common cause of end-stage renal diseases, affecting 30% of T1D patients [97]. GAS6 and its receptor Axl play a key role in the development of glomerular hypertrophy, a hallmark of the early phase of nephropathy. In diabetic rats, it has been demonstrated that GAS6/Axl mediates glomerular hypertrophy during diabetes [96]. However, there is a paucity of information about the association of GAS6 and TLRs, and the involvement of GAS6 as a ligand for TLRs in T1D is unknown. Recently, analyzing the levels of ligands of TLR2 and TLR4 in mononuclear cells isolated from blood samples collected in patients with T1D, Deveraj and coworkers showed increased levels of HSP60 and HMGB1, but no significant difference in the levels of GAS6 between T1D diabetic group and their matched controls [71]. Therefore, further studies are necessary to clarify if there is a link between GAS6 and TLRs in the pathogenesis of T1D.

5. Targeting TLRs to manage T1D

Studies into the mechanisms behind disease progression have tended focus on identifying the important cell types and pathways involved in T1D. Definitely, TLR pathways are involved in T1D, making these receptors a tempting immune-based therapeutic intervention to handle T1D. TLR2 and TLR4 have a potential role in mediating inflammation and consequently, the complications associated with diabetes, mainly vascular damage, making them attractive targets. The deficiency of TLR4 as well as TLR2 is associated with reduced atherosclerosis and inflammatory state in diabetic mice [30, 98]. Treatment with a TLR4 antagonist was shown to inhibit vascular inflammation and atherogenesis in STZ-induced $ApoE^{-/-}$ diabetic mice, as well as lower serum cholesterol and triglyceride levels in nondiabetic $ApoE^{-/-}$ mice [99]. It has been shown that $TLR9^{-/-}$ NOD mice present a delay in the onset of diabetes with decreased IFN-α production and decreased diabetogenic CD8 T cells in pancreatic lymph nodes. Moreover, the addition of a TLR9 antagonist oligodeoxynucleotide or chloroquine inhibited bone-marrow-derived DCs activation and CD8 T cells priming in response to CpG, an agonist of TLR9 [100].

Conversely, TLR agonists have been successfully used in NOD mice to delay T1D by inducing tolerogenic responses [39, 101]. The TLR2 agonist Pam3CSK4, when administered chronically in NOD mice, inhibits the development of T1D. Also, diabetogenic T cell priming of DCs was attenuated by chronic treatment with Pam3CSK4, suggesting DC tolerance [20]. Furthermore, the combination of TLR2 tolerization and inhibition of dipeptydil peptidase 4 (DPP4), which has been demonstrated to ameliorate STZ-induced diabetes by increasing beta-cell mass [102], can reverse early-onset diabetes in NOD mice [101].

Briefly, two contradictory possibilities have been considered regarding TLRs as a target to manage T1D. One is based on the belief that TLRs mediate T1D onset and its complications. Therefore, targeting these receptors using antibody treatment, pharmacological antagonist, or genetic approaches could minimize diabetes complications and decrease inflammation. The second possibility is based on the strategy of inhibiting T1D by tolerance mechanisms. There are scientific reports for both possibilities, making these receptors an attractive future option for treatment of T1D. However, the exact role of TLRs in the pathogenesis of T1D is not completely understood and the initial event of T1D is not revealed. Therefore, therapeutic approaches for T1D using TLR targeting remain a mere theoretical alternative.

6. Conclusion

The idea that the upregulation of TLR pathways, under some circumstances, leads to the induction of proinflammatory responses, and islet destruction is consistent with emerging data in animal models of T1D. In addition, a large body of evidence suggests increased TLR activity in diabetic patients, and these receptors have been suggested to be involved in the pathogenesis of diabetic vasculopathies. Therefore, therapeutic strategies to prevent TLR-mediated inflammation in T1D via modulation of either receptors or their DAMPs ligands can be a welcome addition to the available approaches to deal with T1D and diabetic vascular complications. However, targeting TLRs themselves using approaches such as antagonists could pose the risk of compromising host immunity. In addition, while some antigen-based immunotherapies targeting TLR ligands have proven to be protective against T1D development in animal models, these protocols might not be successfully adaptable to human diabetic patients at the time of diagnosis due to the nature of pathogenic and tolerogenic antigen selection in animal models and human individuals [103].

In fact, there exist number crucial questions regarding TLRs and T1D mechanisms that remain to be addressed. One of the major questions is do TLR pathways promote the initiation or

http://dx.doi.org/10.5772/61925

effector phase of diabetes, or both? A more complete understanding of how the innate immune system via TLRs can modulate autoimmune responses to beta-cell antigens, as well as the mechanisms by which these receptors are contributing to triggering and tuning T1D is crucial, not only because this information can lead to clear elucidation of the role of the innate immune system in TD1 but also because it may clarify whether TLRs can be used as an innovative clinical approach to manage or prevent this disease.

Acknowledgements

Doctor Nunes and Dr. Webb are supported by American Heart Association (Scientific Development Grant, SDG 12080023 and Grant-in-Aid, respectively).

Author details

Kenia Pedrosa Nunes[1*], Eric Guisbert[1], Theodora Szasz[2] and Clinton Webb[2]

*Address all correspondence to: keniapedrosa@gmail.com

1 Department of Biological Sciences, Florida Institute of Technology, Melbourne, FL, USA

2 Department of Physiology, Georgia Regents University, Augusta, GA, USA

References

[1] Janeway, C.A., Jr. and R. Medzhitov, *Innate immune recognition.* Annu Rev Immunol, 2002. 20: p. 197-216.

[2] Meylan, E., J. Tschopp, and M. Karin, *Intracellular pattern recognition receptors in the host response.* Nature, 2006. 442(7098): p. 39-44.

[3] O'Neill, L.A., D. Golenbock, and A.G. Bowie, *The history of Toll-like receptors - redefining innate immunity.* Nat Rev Immunol, 2013. 13(6): p. 453-60.

[4] Lee, C.C., A.M. Avalos, and H.L. Ploegh, *Accessory molecules for Toll-like receptors and their function.* Nat Rev Immunol, 2012. 12(3): p. 168-79.

[5] Assmann, T.S., et al., *Toll-like receptor 3 (TLR3) and the development of type 1 diabetes mellitus.* Arch Endocrinol Metab, 2015. 59(1): p. 4-12.

[6] Devaraj, S., et al., *Increased toll-like receptor (TLR) 2 and TLR4 expression in monocytes from patients with type 1 diabetes: further evidence of a proinflammatory state.* J Clin Endocrinol Metab, 2008. 93(2): p. 578-83.

[7] Schranz, D.B. and A. Lernmark, *Immunology in diabetes: an update.* Diabetes Metab Rev, 1998. 14(1): p. 3-29.

[8] Lien, E. and D. Zipris, *The role of Toll-like receptor pathways in the mechanism of type 1 diabetes.* Curr Mol Med, 2009. 9(1): p. 52-68.

[9] Zipris, D., *Epidemiology of type 1 diabetes and what animal models teach us about the role of viruses in disease mechanisms.* Clin Immunol, 2009. 131(1): p. 11-23.

[10] Todd, J.A., J.I. Bell, and H.O. McDevitt, *HLA-DQ beta gene contributes to susceptibility and resistance to insulin-dependent diabetes mellitus.* Nature, 1987. 329(6140): p. 599-604.

[11] Todd, J.A., et al., *Genetic analysis of autoimmune type 1 diabetes mellitus in mice.* Nature, 1991. 351(6327): p. 542-7.

[12] Rewers, M. and P. Zimmet, *The rising tide of childhood type 1 diabetes--what is the elusive environmental trigger?* Lancet, 2004. 364(9446): p. 1645-7.

[13] Eizirik, D.L. and T. Mandrup-Poulsen, *A choice of death--the signal-transduction of immune-mediated beta-cell apoptosis.* Diabetologia, 2001. 44(12): p. 2115-33.

[14] Komai-Koma, M., et al., *TLR2 is expressed on activated T cells as a costimulatory receptor.* Proc Natl Acad Sci U S A, 2004. 101(9): p. 3029-34.

[15] Jin, B., et al., *The effects of TLR activation on T-cell development and differentiation.* Clin Dev Immunol, 2012. 2012: p. 836485.

[16] Hua, Z. and B. Hou, *TLR signaling in B-cell development and activation.* Cell Mol Immunol, 2013. 10(2): p. 103-6.

[17] Santoni, M., et al., *Toll like receptors and pancreatic diseases: From a pathogenetic mechanism to a therapeutic target.* Cancer Treat Rev, 2015. 41(7): p. 569-76.

[18] Diana, J., et al., *Innate immunity in type 1 diabetes.* Discov Med, 2011. 11(61): p. 513-20.

[19] Lee, M.S., *Role of innate immunity in the pathogenesis of type 1 and type 2 diabetes.* J Korean Med Sci, 2014. 29(8): p. 1038-41.

[20] Lee, M.S., *Treatment of autoimmune diabetes by inhibiting the initial event.* Immune Netw, 2013. 13(5): p. 194-8.

[21] Steinman, R.M., D. Hawiger, and M.C. Nussenzweig, *Tolerogenic dendritic cells.* Annu Rev Immunol, 2003. 21: p. 685-711.

[22] Hammond, T., et al., *Toll-like receptor (TLR) expression on CD4+ and CD8+ T-cells in patients chronically infected with hepatitis C virus.* Cell Immunol, 2010. 264(2): p. 150-5.

[23] Schram, M.T., et al., *Markers of inflammation are cross-sectionally associated with microvascular complications and cardiovascular disease in type 1 diabetes--the EURODIAB Prospective Complications Study.* Diabetologia, 2005. 48(2): p. 370-8.

[24] Devaraj, S., et al., *Evidence of increased inflammation and microcirculatory abnormalities in patients with type 1 diabetes and their role in microvascular complications.* Diabetes, 2007. 56(11): p. 2790-6.

[25] Devaraj, S., et al., *Demonstration of increased toll-like receptor 2 and toll-like receptor 4 expression in monocytes of type 1 diabetes mellitus patients with microvascular complications.* Metabolism, 2011. 60(2): p. 256-9.

[26] Li, H. and B. Sun, *Toll-like receptor 4 in atherosclerosis.* J Cell Mol Med, 2007. 11(1): p. 88-95.

[27] Kayserova, J., et al., *Decreased dendritic cell numbers but increased TLR9-mediated interferon-alpha production in first degree relatives of type 1 diabetes patients.* Clin Immunol, 2014. 153(1): p. 49-55.

[28] Hayashi, T., et al., *Treatment of autoimmune inflammation by a TLR7 ligand regulating the innate immune system.* PLoS One, 2012. 7(9): p. e45860.

[29] Karumuthil-Melethil, S., et al., *TLR2- and Dectin 1-associated innate immune response modulates T-cell response to pancreatic beta-cell antigen and prevents type 1 diabetes.* Diabetes, 2015. 64(4): p. 1341-57.

[30] Devaraj, S., et al., *Knockout of toll-like receptor-2 attenuates both the proinflammatory state of diabetes and incipient diabetic nephropathy.* Arterioscler Thromb Vasc Biol, 2011. 31(8): p. 1796-804.

[31] Sakata, Y., et al., *Toll-like receptor 2 modulates left ventricular function following ischemia-reperfusion injury.* Am J Physiol Heart Circ Physiol, 2007. 292(1): p. H503-9.

[32] Devaraj, S. and I. Jialal, *Increased secretion of IP-10 from monocytes under hyperglycemia is via the TLR2 and TLR4 pathway.* Cytokine, 2009. 47(1): p. 6-10.

[33] Kim, D.H., et al., *Inhibition of autoimmune diabetes by TLR2 tolerance.* J Immunol, 2011. 187(10): p. 5211-20.

[34] Dasu, M.R., et al., *TLR2 expression and signaling-dependent inflammation impair wound healing in diabetic mice.* Lab Invest, 2010. 90(11): p. 1628-36.

[35] Mudaliar, H., et al., *The role of TLR2 and 4-mediated inflammatory pathways in endothelial cells exposed to high glucose.* PLoS One, 2014. 9(10): p. e108844.

[36] Shigihara, T., et al., *Significance of serum CXCL10/IP-10 level in type 1 diabetes.* J Autoimmun, 2006. 26(1): p. 66-71.

[37] Caramalho, I., et al., *Regulatory T cells selectively express toll-like receptors and are activated by lipopolysaccharide.* J Exp Med, 2003. 197(4): p. 403-11.

[38] Liu, H., et al., *Toll-like receptor 2 signaling modulates the functions of CD4+ CD25+ regulatory T cells.* Proc Natl Acad Sci U S A, 2006. 103(18): p. 7048-53.

[39] Filippi, C.M., et al., *TLR2 signaling improves immunoregulation to prevent type 1 diabetes.* Eur J Immunol, 2011. 41(5): p. 1399-409.

[40] Wen, L., et al., *Innate immunity and intestinal microbiota in the development of Type 1 diabetes.* Nature, 2008. 455(7216): p. 1109-13.

[41] Kachapati, K., et al., *The non-obese diabetic (NOD) mouse as a model of human type 1 diabetes.* Methods Mol Biol, 2012. 933: p. 3-16.

[42] Kim, H.S., et al., *Toll-like receptor 2 senses beta-cell death and contributes to the initiation of autoimmune diabetes.* Immunity, 2007. 27(2): p. 321-33.

[43] Gulden, E., et al., *Toll-like receptor 4 deficiency accelerates the development of insulin-deficient diabetes in non-obese diabetic mice.* PLoS One, 2013. 8(9): p. e75385.

[44] Dong, B., et al., *TLR4 regulates cardiac lipid accumulation and diabetic heart disease in the nonobese diabetic mouse model of type 1 diabetes.* Am J Physiol Heart Circ Physiol, 2012. 303(6): p. H732-42.

[45] Bednar, K.J. and W.M. Ridgway, *Targeting innate immunity for treatment of type 1 diabetes.* Immunotherapy, 2014. 6(12): p. 1239-42.

[46] Bednar, K.J., et al., *Reversal of New-Onset Type 1 Diabetes with an agonistic TLR4/MD-2 Monoclonal Antibody.* Diabetes, 2015.

[47] Vallois, D., et al., *The type 1 diabetes locus Idd6 controls TLR1 expression.* J Immunol, 2007. 179(6): p. 3896-903.

[48] Assmann, T.S., et al., *Polymorphisms in the TLR3 gene are associated with risk for type 1 diabetes mellitus.* Eur J Endocrinol, 2014. 170(4): p. 519-27.

[49] Pirie, F.J., et al., *Toll-like receptor 3 gene polymorphisms in South African Blacks with type 1 diabetes.* Tissue Antigens, 2005. 66(2): p. 125-30.

[50] Coppieters, K.T., T. Boettler, and M. von Herrath, *Virus infections in type 1 diabetes.* Cold Spring Harb Perspect Med, 2012. 2(1): p. a007682.

[51] Lee, A.S., et al., *Toll-like receptor 7 stimulation promotes autoimmune diabetes in the NOD mouse.* Diabetologia, 2011. 54(6): p. 1407-16.

[52] Hayashi, T., et al., *Induction of Tolerogenic Dendritic Cells by a PEGylated TLR7 Ligand for Treatment of Type 1 Diabetes.* PLoS One, 2015. 10(6): p. e0129867.

[53] Zipris, D., et al., *TLR9-signaling pathways are involved in Kilham rat virus-induced autoimmune diabetes in the biobreeding diabetes-resistant rat.* J Immunol, 2007. 178(2): p. 693-701.

[54] Edfeldt, K., et al., *Expression of toll-like receptors in human atherosclerotic lesions: a possible pathway for plaque activation.* Circulation, 2002. 105(10): p. 1158-61.

[55] Curtiss, L.K. and P.S. Tobias, *Emerging role of Toll-like receptors in atherosclerosis.* J Lipid Res, 2009. 50 Suppl: p. S340-5.

[56] Swerdlow, A.J. and M.E. Jones, *Mortality during 25 years of follow-up of a cohort with diabetes.* Int J Epidemiol, 1996. 25(6): p. 1250-61.

[57] Soedamah-Muthu, S.S., et al., *High risk of cardiovascular disease in patients with type 1 diabetes in the U.K.: a cohort study using the general practice research database.* Diabetes Care, 2006. 29(4): p. 798-804.

[58] Chait, A. and K.E. Bornfeldt, *Diabetes and atherosclerosis: is there a role for hyperglycemia?* J Lipid Res, 2009. 50 Suppl: p. S335-9.

[59] Yung, L.M., et al., *Reactive oxygen species in vascular wall.* Cardiovasc Hematol Disord Drug Targets, 2006. 6(1): p. 1-19.

[60] Asehnoune, K., et al., *Involvement of reactive oxygen species in Toll-like receptor 4-dependent activation of NF-kappa B.* J Immunol, 2004. 172(4): p. 2522-9.

[61] Chen, J.X. and A. Stinnett, *Critical role of the NADPH oxidase subunit p47phox on vascular TLR expression and neointimal lesion formation in high-fat diet-induced obesity.* Lab Invest, 2008. 88(12): p. 1316-28.

[62] Rajamani, U. and I. Jialal, *Hyperglycemia induces Toll-like receptor-2 and -4 expression and activity in human microvascular retinal endothelial cells: implications for diabetic retinopathy.* J Diabetes Res, 2014. 2014: p. 790902.

[63] Shin, J.J., et al., *Damage-associated molecular patterns and their pathological relevance in diabetes mellitus.* Ageing Res Rev, 2015.

[64] Lotze, M.T. and K.J. Tracey, *High-mobility group box 1 protein (HMGB1): nuclear weapon in the immune arsenal.* Nat Rev Immunol, 2005. 5(4): p. 331-42.

[65] Wang, H., H. Yang, and K.J. Tracey, *Extracellular role of HMGB1 in inflammation and sepsis.* J Intern Med, 2004. 255(3): p. 320-31.

[66] Tang, D., et al., *High-mobility group box 1, oxidative stress, and disease.* Antioxid Redox Signal, 2011. 14(7): p. 1315-35.

[67] Lotze, M.T., A. Deisseroth, and A. Rubartelli, *Damage associated molecular pattern molecules.* Clin Immunol, 2007. 124(1): p. 1-4.

[68] Nogueira-Machado, J.A., et al., *HMGB1, TLR and RAGE: a functional tripod that leads to diabetic inflammation.* Expert Opin Ther Targets, 2011. 15(8): p. 1023-35.

[69] Park, J.S., et al., *High mobility group box 1 protein interacts with multiple Toll-like receptors.* Am J Physiol Cell Physiol, 2006. 290(3): p. C917-24.

[70] Branco-Madeira, F. and B.N. Lambrecht, *High mobility group box-1 recognition: the beginning of a RAGEless era?* EMBO Mol Med, 2010. 2(6): p. 193-5.

[71] Devaraj, S., et al., *Increased levels of ligands of Toll-like receptors 2 and 4 in type 1 diabetes.* Diabetologia, 2009. 52(8): p. 1665-8.

[72] Li, M., et al., *Toll-like receptor 4 on islet beta cells senses expression changes in high-mobility group box 1 and contributes to the initiation of type 1 diabetes.* Exp Mol Med, 2012. 44(4): p. 260-7.

[73] Dasu, M.R., et al., *Increased toll-like receptor (TLR) activation and TLR ligands in recently diagnosed type 2 diabetic subjects.* Diabetes Care, 2010. 33(4): p. 861-8.

[74] Li, J., et al., *Recombinant HMGB1 with cytokine-stimulating activity.* J Immunol Methods, 2004. 289(1-2): p. 211-23.

[75] Dandona, P., et al., *Insulin infusion suppresses while glucose infusion induces Toll-like receptors and high-mobility group-B1 protein expression in mononuclear cells of type 1 diabetes patients.* Am J Physiol Endocrinol Metab, 2013. 304(8): p. E810-8.

[76] Schlueter, C., et al., *Angiogenetic signaling through hypoxia: HMGB1: an angiogenetic switch molecule.* Am J Pathol, 2005. 166(4): p. 1259-63.

[77] Biscetti, F., et al., *High-mobility group box-1 protein promotes angiogenesis after peripheral ischemia in diabetic mice through a VEGF-dependent mechanism.* Diabetes, 2010. 59(6): p. 1496-505.

[78] Lin, Q., et al., *High-mobility group box-1 mediates toll-like receptor 4-dependent angiogenesis.* Arterioscler Thromb Vasc Biol, 2011. 31(5): p. 1024-32.

[79] van Beijnum, J.R., et al., *Gene expression of tumor angiogenesis dissected: specific targeting of colon cancer angiogenic vasculature.* Blood, 2006. 108(7): p. 2339-48.

[80] Porto, A., et al., *Smooth muscle cells in human atherosclerotic plaques secrete and proliferate in response to high mobility group box 1 protein.* FASEB J, 2006. 20(14): p. 2565-6.

[81] Guisbert, E., et al., *Identification of a tissue-selective heat shock response regulatory network.* PLoS Genet, 2013. 9(4): p. e1003466.

[82] Tsan, M.F. and B. Gao, *Heat shock proteins and immune system.* J Leukoc Biol, 2009. 85(6): p. 905-10.

[83] Asea, A., *Heat shock proteins and toll-like receptors.* Handb Exp Pharmacol, 2008(183): p. 111-27.

[84] Abulafia-Lapid, R., et al., *T cells and autoantibodies to human HSP70 in type 1 diabetes in children.* J Autoimmun, 2003. 20(4): p. 313-21.

[85] Abulafia-Lapid, R., et al., *T cell proliferative responses of type 1 diabetes patients and healthy individuals to human hsp60 and its peptides.* J Autoimmun, 1999. 12(2): p. 121-9.

[86] Birk, O.S., et al., *NOD mouse diabetes: the ubiquitous mouse hsp60 is a beta-cell target antigen of autoimmune T cells.* J Autoimmun, 1996. 9(2): p. 159-66.

[87] Krause, M., et al., *Elevated levels of extracellular heat-shock protein 72 (eHSP72) are positively correlated with insulin resistance in vivo and cause pancreatic beta-cell dysfunction and death in vitro.* Clin Sci (Lond), 2014. 126(10): p. 739-52.

[88] Bockova, J., D. Elias, and I.R. Cohen, *Treatment of NOD diabetes with a novel peptide of the hsp60 molecule induces Th2-type antibodies.* J Autoimmun, 1997. 10(4): p. 323-9.

[89] Raz, I., et al., *Treatment of new-onset type 1 diabetes with peptide DiaPep277 is safe and associated with preserved beta-cell function: extension of a randomized, double-blind, phase II trial.* Diabetes Metab Res Rev, 2007. 23(4): p. 292-8.

[90] Raz, I., et al., *Beta-cell function in new-onset type 1 diabetes and immunomodulation with a heat-shock protein peptide (DiaPep277): a randomised, double-blind, phase II trial.* Lancet, 2001. 358(9295): p. 1749-53.

[91] *Treatment of recent-onset type 1 diabetic patients with DiaPep277: results of a double-blind, placebo-controlled, randomized phase 3 trial. Diabetes Care 2014;37:1392-1400. DOI: 10.2337/dc13-1391.* Diabetes Care, 2015. 38(1): p. 178.

[92] Raz, I., et al., *Treatment of recent-onset type 1 diabetic patients with DiaPep277: results of a double-blind, placebo-controlled, randomized phase 3 trial.* Diabetes Care, 2014. 37(5): p. 1392-400.

[93] Rajaiah, R. and K.D. Moudgil, *Heat-shock proteins can promote as well as regulate autoimmunity.* Autoimmun Rev, 2009. 8(5): p. 388-93.

[94] Noble, E.G. and G.X. Shen, *Impact of exercise and metabolic disorders on heat shock proteins and vascular inflammation.* Autoimmune Dis, 2012. 2012: p. 836519.

[95] Qu, B., et al., *The detection and role of heat shock protein 70 in various nondisease conditions and disease conditions: a literature review.* Cell Stress Chaperones, 2015.

[96] Nagai, K., et al., *Growth arrest-specific gene 6 is involved in glomerular hypertrophy in the early stage of diabetic nephropathy.* J Biol Chem, 2003. 278(20): p. 18229-34.

[97] Bojestig, M., et al., *Declining incidence of nephropathy in insulin-dependent diabetes mellitus.* N Engl J Med, 1994. 330(1): p. 15-8.

[98] Devaraj, S., P. Tobias, and I. Jialal, *Knockout of toll-like receptor-4 attenuates the pro-inflammatory state of diabetes.* Cytokine, 2011. 55(3): p. 441-5.

[99] Lu, Z., et al., *TLR4 antagonist reduces early-stage atherosclerosis in diabetic apolipoprotein E-deficient mice.* J Endocrinol, 2013. 216(1): p. 61-71.

[100] Zhang, Y., et al., *TLR9 blockade inhibits activation of diabetogenic CD8+ T cells and delays autoimmune diabetes.* J Immunol, 2010. 184(10): p. 5645-53.

[101] Kim, D.H., et al., *Treatment of autoimmune diabetes in NOD mice by Toll-like receptor 2 tolerance in conjunction with dipeptidyl peptidase 4 inhibition.* Diabetologia, 2012. 55(12): p. 3308-17.

[102] Cho, J.M., et al., *A novel dipeptidyl peptidase IV inhibitor DA-1229 ameliorates streptozotocin-induced diabetes by increasing beta-cell replication and neogenesis.* Diabetes Res Clin Pract, 2011. 91(1): p. 72-9.

[103] Serreze, D.V. and Y.G. Chen, *Of mice and men: use of animal models to identify possible interventions for the prevention of autoimmune type 1 diabetes in humans.* Trends Immunol, 2005. 26(11): p. 603-7.

Chapter 2

The Pancreas Secreting Insulin for Decades after Onset of Type I Diabetes — Implications for Care and Management

Denise L. Faustman and Miriam Davis

Additional information is available at the end of the chapter

http://dx.doi.org/10.5772/61234

Abstract

Up until recently, the prevailing dogma was that insulin secretion ceased within a couple of years after the diagnosis of type I diabetes, a clinical time period called the honeymoon. But a series of recent studies have established that release of C-peptide, which is the best measure of endogenous insulin production, can commonly persist for decades after disease onset. The release of C-peptide, even at low levels, is shown to have functional and clinical significance. For example, C-peptide levels >10 pmol/l are associated with fewer diabetes complications, i.e., nephropathy, neuropathy, foot ulcers, and retinopathy. The diabetic population may also be heterogeneous in risk for fall in C-peptide, with early age of diabetes onset a risk factor for more rapid C-peptide decline. The persistence of insulin release for decades and its functional and clinical significance suggest that assays for C-peptide should be a regular part of diabetes management. Furthermore, patients with established diabetes should be eligible to participate in clinical trials of immune therapies since preservation of these low levels appears clinically important to prevent complications.

Keywords: Type 1 diabetes, C-peptide, insulin secretion, complications

1. Introduction

1.1. Background

The reigning view of the type I diabetes field had been until recently that the pancreas commonly stops secreting insulin within a number of years of diagnosis. The so-called honeymoon period post disease onset has been explained to patients since the seminal publication in 1986 by George Eisenbarth on the natural history of diabetes [1]. After the honeymoon period, patients were cautioned to expect that their pancreas was functionally inactive as it related to insulin secretion and could no longer be saved. An iconic image depicting the rapid demise of islet function as measured by C-peptide, which is cosecreted with insulin, has been a staple for teaching medical students and in continuing education courses for physicians. And the consequence of the honeymoon period has been that patients with established disease are routinely excluded from immune intervention trials. Most, if not all, immunotherapy trials conducted over the past 20 years have excluded all but new-onset cases of type 1 diabetes under the assumption that the pancreas was not salvageable if the disease was past the honeymoon period and all insulin secretion has ceased. Indeed, the current definition of type 1 diabetes by the American Diabetes Association (ADA) is a disease leading to "absolute insulin deficiency" [2].

Despite this dogma, there were clues questioning the view that the pancreas of type 1 diabetics ceases function within a short number of years after diagnosis. There had been histological indications that the islets were not uniformly dead dating back as early as 1902. The pathologist M.B. Schmidt documented the rare existence of intact islet-like structures in an autopsy of a child with type I diabetes [3]. Decades later, several other studies from 1959 to 1985 also documented histologically the existence of occasional intact islet cells among patients at all stages of disease [3-8]. More recent confirmation of histologically intact islet cells comes from several studies [9-12]. Nevertheless, these studies did not prompt questioning of the short honeymoon period because the evidence was only histologic and not accompanied by functional studies. It was thought by the majority that if the insulin-secreting structures could be found they lacked functional insulin secretion since it could not be detected.

An early indication of long-term persistence of insulin release was present in 2008 with an immune interventional trial that compared long-term diabetic serum samples in the traditional C-peptide assays compared to newer more sensitive C-peptide assays. C-peptide assays are the best measures of endogenous insulin secretion. C-peptide is cosecreted with insulin in equimolar amounts by the pancreatic beta-islet cells upon enzymatic cleavage of the prohormone precursor proinsulin. C-peptide is more advantageous to measure than insulin because it is unaffected by exogenous insulin treatment, and because the liver metabolizes much of the insulin secreted into the portal vein, but negligibly metabolizes C-peptide. Insulin's high metabolism by the liver means that peripheral insulin levels may not best reflect portal insulin secretion. C-peptide is also advantageous because its half-life is longer than that of insulin, circulating systemically at concentrations about five times higher. Low C-peptide can be used to distinguish type 1 from type 2 diabetes, the latter marked by high levels of C-peptide early in disease [13].

The immune interventional trial of Bovine Calmette Guerin (BCG) in diabetic patients with established disease (a mean of 15 years) [14] studied fasting and stimulated C-peptides over a 2-year period. A condition of enrollment in the trial was that there was no fasting or stimulated C-peptide as measured by traditional C-peptide assay whose lower limit of detection is about 50 pmol/l. To the surprise of all, at the end of the trial all serum was restudied for C-peptide, this time using ultrasensitive C-peptide assay. All long-term recipients of the immunotherapy, as well as placebo patients, had low yet detectable levels of C-peptide at baseline both as fasting and stimulated and throughout the course of the trial.

2. Persistence and functional significance of C-peptide

This unexpected finding motivated a systematic study of C-peptide levels in 182 diabetic patients using the ultrasensitive assay. Glycemic levels were also evaluated in a subset of patients—with normoglycemia at <150 mg/dl and hyperglycemia at >150 mg/dl. Samples from hyperglycemic patients had significantly higher C-peptide levels than those with normoglycemia [15]. The study found a linear relationship between glycemic levels and C-peptide, indicating intact islet-cell functioning because higher glycemic levels stimulate release of insulin. Islet-cell function was intact at C-peptide levels as meager as 2.8 pmol/l. These analyses revealed that despite low levels of C-peptide, some islet-cell function remains decades after diagnosis. The release of C-peptide was analyzed according to 5-year disease duration intervals. C-peptide was found above limits of detection in patients with up to 40 years of disease duration (Figure 1). As duration increased, C-peptide levels tended to gradually decline over decades. In order of increasing duration, C-peptide was higher than the detection limit at rates of 78.9% (0-5 years duration), 59.5% (6-10 years duration), 39.5% (11-20 years duration), 39.1% (21-30 years duration), 10% (31-40 years duration), and 0% (>40 years duration). Thus, longer disease duration is related to lower levels of C-peptide production. The long-term persistence of C-peptide release contradicts the traditional model that C-peptide disappears 1-2 years or a short time after diagnosis and contradicts the ADA definition of type 1 diabetes as an absolute deficiency of insulin. Also, it was reported that type 1 diabetics with early age of onset had a faster decay of C-peptide; type 1 diabetics with later onset of diabetes had slower declines in C-peptide. This suggested that there was age-of-onset variability in the diabetic population as related to total loss of pancreas function.

A study by Oram and colleagues [16] soon followed and confirmed the long-term persistence of C-peptide secretion as measured by stimulated urine studies. Studying 74 volunteers, they found that 73% of patients with type I diabetes of more than 5 years duration (median 29 years) had detectable C-peptide as measured by electrochemiluminescence assay (detection limit 3.3 pmol/l). To study function, the investigators conducted a mixed-meal tolerance test. C-peptide levels either rose (n=43) or remained the same (n=11) in response to a meal in all patients with detectable serum C-peptide in urine. The study concluded that most diabetics with long-term disease continue to produce low levels of insulin and that a small number of islet cells are still functional, suggesting that these cells are escaping immune attack or are regenerating. This study was also of note since the measurement of remaining C-peptide was performed using a different C-peptide assay from Wang and colleagues, thus decreasing the chance that these early reports of persistent C-peptide secretion were an artifact of the improved C-peptide monitoring techniques and assays.

Three other investigative teams, reporting in abstract form, uncovered evidence of the long-term persistence of C-peptide production in early 2014. Two of the studies also found increased

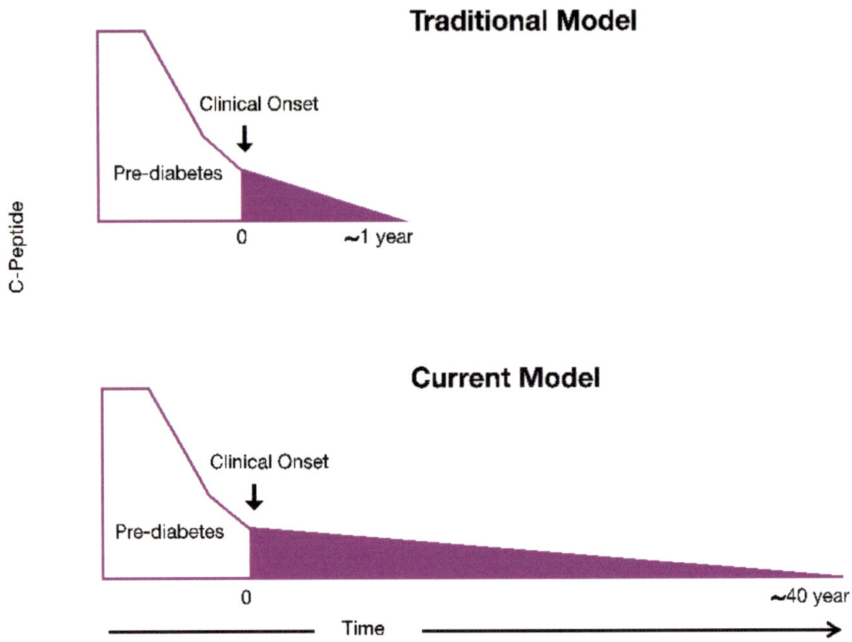

Figure 1. The traditional model of type 1 diabetes predicts the pancreas will stop producing C-peptide within a short time after disease onset, typically 1-3 years. New data now show that a typical course of type 1 diabetes is the long-term persistence of C-peptide for decades in many type 1 diabetic subjects.

output of C-peptide after a mixed-meal tolerance test [17, 18]. The third study was large: it recruited 944 patients in a population-based study design, finding insulin secretion in long-duration type 1 diabetics, but the study did not examine islet-cell function [19].

More recently, in late 2014, the rapidly expanding literature confirmed the frequent and long-term persistence of C-peptide for decades after the onset of type 1 diabetes. McGee and colleagues evaluated whether clinically relevant concentrations of stimulated C-peptide can be detected after 30 years in the Diabetes Control and Complications Trial (DCCT) cohorts. Studying 58 participants, 17% of the enrolled subjects had a definitive response with stimulated C-peptide greater than 30 pmol/L [20]. Using nonfasting random C-peptides, Davis and colleagues detected 29% of 919 individuals with remaining C-peptide with a lower limit of sensitivity of 20 pmol/L in a C-peptide assay [21].

What protects or places at risk type 1 diabetic subjects for improved preservation of C-peptide? In 1978, Madsbad and colleagues reported on the prevalence of residual beta cell function in insulin-dependent diabetics in relation to age of onset and duration (21). In 1987, two research groups found similar associations of early age of onset associated with faster decay of C-peptide immediately after diabetes onset [22, 23]. Wang and colleagues, using C-peptide assays with lower limits of detection to 2.5 pmol/L combined with a decades-long evaluation of the full disease course, confirmed that age of onset was related to long-term preservation for up to 40 years after diagnosis [15]. Ludvigsson and colleagues studied the decline of C-peptide during the first year after diagnosis of type 1 children and adolescents and reported a faster decline of C-peptide in younger subjects [24]. Barker and colleagues, in a large 3,668 subject study for 5 years after diagnosis, more recently demonstrated age at diagnosis of type 1 diabetes was a strong correlate of a more rapid decline of C-peptide function, with young children again losing pancreas insulin secretion at more rapid rates [25]. Therefore, a very clear protective factor for a slow C-peptide decay is older age of onset, and a very clear risk factor for rapid decline in C-peptide is younger age of onset. The only exception to this reproducible trend is with age of onset of diabetes greater than 40 years of age: C-peptide again starts to decay faster and these subjects are also notable for the majority having long-standing hypothyroidism prior to diabetes onset [15].

Should it have been known earlier that the ADA definition of "absolute insulin deficiency" of type 1 diabetes was wrong, especially as it relates to residual C-peptide over decades, not just variable fall in C-peptide close to onset? It was known from the Joslin 50-year Medalist Study that some fortunate type 1 diabetics that lived for at least 50 years with this disease were also blessed with random C-peptide levels greater than 30 pmol/L [12]. Still it was viewed that these very fortunate type 1 diabetics were the exception. These data reinforced early the concept that residual C-peptide was associated with better HbA1c and longevity. Again, using less sensitive assays with cutoff values of 40-50 pmol/L it was known from the DCCT that only 11% of patients screened by stimulated C-peptide measurements had any C-peptide at 2 years after diagnosis [26]. As mentioned earlier, for nearly 100 years histologic studies had uncovered islet-like structures consistent with the insulin-secreting cells of the pancreas, but without accompanying functional data of insulin secretion it was difficult to interpret the findings.

3. Do low levels of C-peptide have clinical significance?

Low levels of C-peptide may be produced but do they have any clinical significance? The answer to the question is a resounding yes, according to recently study that was published [27]. First, the 8-year study replicated—in a much larger sample (n = 1273) than an earlier study—the findings that the pancreas continued to produce C-peptide for decades after diagnosis was confirmed. The study also found that fasting C-peptide output, above as low as 10 pmol/L, is associated with fewer diabetes-related complications (e.g., nephropathy, neuropathy, and cardiovascular disease). Low levels of C-peptide were also associated with poorer metabolic control, as captured by HbA1c. The study found that the lowest levels of C-peptide were associated with severe hypoglycemia. Finally, all levels of measurable C-peptide were responsive to fluctuations in blood glucose levels as assessed by 1,5-Anhydroglucitol, a marker responsive to glucose fluctuations. This study complements the work of Lachin and colleagues that restudied the DCCT subjects, albeit with older C-peptide assays with less sensitivity and lower limits of sensitivity to 40-50 pmol/L [28]. Regardless, both fasting and stimulated C-peptide remaining levels were associated in a linear manner to prevention of complications. This resulted in a conclusion that preservations of stimulated C-peptide greater than 200 pmol/L has clinical benefit. The Kuhtreiber study suggests that preservation of fasting C-peptide to the new lower limits of detection of 2.5 pmol/L is even clinically significant.

The studies finding the long-term persistence of C-peptide help to interpret two puzzling scientific observations published more than 15 years ago. The first observation was in identical twins who were discordant for type I diabetes for greater than 20 years who received a hemi-pancreas transplant from the identical twin [29]. Within several weeks, the half-pancreas transplant from the healthy twin to the diabetic twin failed. This was unexpected, because transplants normally are rejected after years, not weeks. The fact that the diabetic twin mounted an aggressive autoimmune response decades after disease onset and after the pancreas was thought to be dead indicates functional islet cells still capable of provoking an autoimmune response. The second observation related to B-lymphocytes: 67% of patients with disease duration of 10 years were positive for at least one diabetes-associated autoantibody and 42% of patients tested positive for 2 to 3 autoantibodies [30]. This finding can now be explained by a primed immune cell attack against residual islet-cell regeneration or long-term survival.

4. Conclusions

The weight of the evidence from several recent studies now points to viable and functional islet cells in long-term type 1 diabetes and should refute therapeutic nihilism that, after a short time after diagnosis, most type 1 diabetics have a pancreas that can no longer produce any insulin. Instead, low-level insulin release can commonly persist for decades after disease onset and has functional and clinical significance. Insulin release is best measured by C-peptide, which is cosecreted with insulin by the beta cells in the islets. C-peptide is preferable to studying remaining insulin secretion because it is unaffected by exogenous insulin treatment and now more sensitive assays allow better limits of detection. Maintenance of even low levels of C-peptide is associated with fewer diabetic complications, better metabolic control (as captured by HbA1c), and is associated with less severe hypoglycemia. The functional and clinical significance of even low levels of C-peptide release suggests that patients should be monitored routinely for C-peptide output combined with other clinical monitors of residual insulin production. The evidence of viable and functional islet cells decades after diagnosis of type 1 diabetes and their protection against diabetic complications also suggest that patients with long-standing disease should not be excluded from immunotherapy clinical trials.

Author details

Denise L. Faustman[1,2*] and Miriam Davis[1]

*Address all correspondence to: faustman@helix.mgh.harvard.edu

1 Immunobiology Laboratory, Massachusetts General Hospital, Boston, MA, USA

2 Harvard Medical School, Boston, MA, USA

References

[1] Eisenbarth GS (1986) Type I diabetes mellitus: a chronic autoimmune disease. *New Engl J Med.* 314: 1360-1368.

[2] American Diabetes A (2014) Standards of medical care in diabetes–2014. *Diabetes Care* 37 Suppl 1: S14-S80.

[3] Schmidt MB (1902) Uber die Beziehung der Langerhans' schen Inseln des Pankreas zum Diabetes Mellitus. *Munch med Wochenschr* 49: 51-54.

[4] Maclean N and Ogilvie RF (1959) Observations on the pancreatic islet tissue of young diabetic subjects. *Diabetes* 8: 83-91.

[5] Gepts W (1965) Pathologic anatomy of the pancreas in juvenile diabetes mellitus. *Diabetes* 14: 619-33.

[6] Doniach I and Morgan AG (1973) Islets of Langerhans in juvenile diabetes mellitus. *Clin Endocrinol* (*Oxf*) 2: 233-48.

[7] Junker K, Egeberg J, Kromann H and Nerup J (1977) An autopsy study of the islets of Langerhans in acute-onset juvenile diabetes mellitus. *Acta Pathol Microbiol Scand A* 85: 699-706.

[8] Foulis A (1985) Autumn Books: Bernard on le pancreas. *Br Med J* (*Clin Res Ed*) 291: 1182.

[9] Meier JJ, Bhushan A, Butler AE, Rizza RA and Butler PC (2005) Sustained beta cell apoptosis in patients with long-standing type 1 diabetes: indirect evidence for islet regeneration? *Diabetologia* 48: 2221-8.

[10] Willcox A, Richardson SJ, Bone AJ, Foulis AK and Morgan NG (2009) Analysis of islet inflammation in human type 1 diabetes. *Clin Exp Immunol* 155: 173-81.

[11] Atkinson MA and Gianani R (2009) The pancreas in human type 1 diabetes: providing new answers to age-old questions. *Curr Opin Endocrinol Diabetes Obes* 16: 279-85.

[12] Keenan HA, Sun JK, Levine J, Doria A, Aiello LP, Eisenbarth G, Bonner-Weir S and King GL (2010) Residual insulin production and pancreatic ss-cell turnover after 50 years of diabetes: Joslin Medalist Study. *Diabetes* 59: 2846-53.

[13] Jones AG and Hattersley AT (2013) The clinical utility of C-peptide measurement in the care of patients with diabetes. *Diabet Med* 30: 803-17.

[14] Faustman DL, Wang L, Okubo Y, Burger D, Ban L, Man G, Zheng H, Schoenfeld D, Pompei R, Avruch J and Nathan DM (2012) Proof-of-concept, randomized, controlled clinical trial of Bacillus-Calmette-Guerin for treatment of long-term type 1 diabetes. *PLoS One* 7: e41756.

[15] Wang L, Lovejoy NF and Faustman DL (2012) Persistence of prolonged C-peptide production in type 1 diabetes as measured with an ultrasensitive C-peptide assay. *Diabetes Care* 35: 465-70.

[16] Oram RA, Jones AG, Besser RE, Knight BA, Shields BM, Brown RJ, Hattersley AT and McDonald TJ (2014) The majority of patients with long-duration type 1 diabetes are insulin microsecretors and have functioning beta cells. *Diabetologia* 57: 187-91.

[17] Bingley PJ, Aitken RJ, Wilson IV, Long AE, Williams AJK, McDonald TJ, Wong S, Hattersley AT and Gillespie KM (2014) Residual beta cell function in long-standing childhood onset type 1 diabetes. *Diabetologia* 57: S189-S190.

[18] Tamer G, Dogan B, Ocakoglu I, Kostek O, Kartal I, Sagun G, Adas M, Tamer I, Mutlu HH and Orhun A (2014) Functioning beta cells in type 1 diabetes may not be as low as it is presumed. *Diabetologia* 57: S189.

[19] McDonald TJ, Oram R, Shields B, Pearson E and Hattersley A (2014) Most people with long duration of type 1 diabetes are insulin microsecretors and produce their own endogenous insulin. *Diabetologia* S510:

[20] McGee P, Steffes M, Nowicki M, Bayless M, Gubitosi-Klug R, Cleary P, Lachin J, Palmer J and Group DER (2014) Insulin secretion measured by stimulated C-peptide in long-established Type 1 diabetes in the Diabetes Control and Complications Trial (DCCT)/ Epidemiology of Diabetes Interventions and Complications (EDIC) cohort: a pilot study. *Diabet Med* 31: 1264-8.

[21] Davis AK, DuBose SN, Haller MJ, Miller KM, DiMeglio LA, Bethin KE, Goland RS, Greenberg EM, Liljenquist DR, Ahmann AJ, Marcovina SM, Peters AL, Beck RW, Greenbaum CJ and for the TDECN (2015) Prevalence of detectable C-peptide according to age at diagnosis and duration of Type 1 diabetes. *Diabetes Care* 38:476-81

[22] DCCT (1987) Effects of age, duration and treatment of insulin-dependent diabetes mellitus on residual beta-cell function: observations during eligibility testing for the Diabetes Control and Complications Trial (DCCT). *J Clin Endocrinol Metab* 65: 30-6.

[23] Giordano C, Galluzzo A, Panto F, Caruso C and Bompiani G (1987) Prevalence of residual B-cell function related to age at onet and genetic profile in newly diagnosed type 1 diabetics. *Acta Diabetol* 24: 317-323.

[24] Ludvigsson J, Carlsson A, Deli A, Forsander G, Ivarsson SA, Kockum I, Lindblad B, Marcus C, Lernmark A and Samuelsson U (2013) Decline of C-peptide during the first year after diagnosis of Type 1 diabetes in children and adolescents. *Diabetes Res Clin Pract* 100: 203-9.

[25] Barker A, Lauria A, Schloot N, Hosszufalusi N, Ludvigsson J, Mathieu C, Mauricio D, Nordwall M, Van der Schueren B, Mandrup-Poulsen T, Scherbaum WA, Weets I, Gorus FK, Wareham N, Leslie RD and Pozzilli P (2014) Age-dependent decline of be-

ta-cell function in type 1 diabetes after diagnosis: a multi-centre longitudinal study. *Diabetes Obes Metab* 16: 262-7.

[26] Steffes MW, Sibley S, Jackson M and Thomas W (2003) Beta-cell function and the development of diabetes-related complications in the diabetes control and complications trial. *Diabetes Care* 26: 832-6.

[27] Faustman DL, Kuhtreiber WM, Washer SLL, Hsu E, Zhao M, Reinhold PE, Burger DE and Zheng H., Faustman DL (2015) Low levels of C-peptide production protect from complications and improve HbA1c control in long-standing type 1 diabetes. Diabetic Medicine DOI: 10.1111/dme.12850.

[28] Lachin JM, McGee P, Palmer JP and Group DER (2014) Impact of C-peptide preservation on metabolic and clinical outcomes in the Diabetes Control and Complications Trial. *Diabetes* 63: 739-48.

[29] Sutherland DE, Sibley R, Xu XZ, Micheal A, Srikanta AM, Taub F, Najarian J and Goetz FC (1984) Twin-to-twin pancreas transplantation: reversal and reenactment of the pathogenesis of type I diabetes. *Trans Assoc Am Phys* 97: 80-87.

[30] Savola K, Sabbah E, Kulmala P, Vahasalo P, Ilonen J and Knip M (1998) Autoantibodies associated with Type I diabetes mellitus persist after diagnosis in children. Diabetologia 41: 1293-7.

Chapter 3

Management of Diabetic Retinopathy and Other Ocular Complications in Type 1 Diabetes

Efraim Berco, Daniel Rappoport, Ayala Pollack, Guy Kleinmann and Yoel Greenwald

Additional information is available at the end of the chapter

http://dx.doi.org/10.5772/61276

Abstract

Type 1 diabetes can reduce vision by affecting various parts of the eye. Proactive, interdisciplinary coordination of treatment and timely referrals can aid in the minimization of visually threatening complications, significantly enhancing patient quality of life. The main causes of visual impairment in diabetes are proliferative diabetic retinopathy and macular edema. Until recently, the mainstay of treatment for both conditions was retinal laser, which prevented significant vision loss but was much less effective at improving vision, especially in macular edema. Over the past decade, exciting new advances in treating diabetic eye disease, namely intraocular steroid and antivascular endothelial growth factor injections, have greatly improved the visual prognosis for the majority of patients with diabetic eye disease.

Keywords: Diabetic retinopathy, Macular edema, Laser, Intraocular injection, Cataract

1. Introduction

Type 1 diabetes is a complex metabolic disease that involves multiple organ systems which can cause severe visual impairment. Almost all ocular structures may be afflicted in diabetes including: the extraocular muscles, the intraocular lens, the optic nerve, and the retina.

Diabetes is the leading cause of blindness between the ages of 20 and 74 in many developed countries. Individuals with diabetes are 25 times more likely to become legally blind than individuals without diabetes. The aspect of diabetic eye disease most responsible for vision loss is diabetic retinopathy, which accounts for ¼ of blind registrations in the Western world [1,2]. There are two main pathways by which diabetic retinopathy affects vision; fluid accumulation in the center of vision, or macular edema, and the formation of pathological retinal vessels also known as proliferative diabetic retinopathy.

Prevention of severe visual impairment in type 1 diabetes includes: optimal glycemic control, the treatment of ancillary risk factors such as hypertension, and regular screening for early diagnosis and treatment of ocular complications.

In the following chapter, we will describe how diabetes affects different ocular structures and discuss the treatment options available today to combat these complications.

2. Extraocular muscles

Patients with diabetes may present with a sudden onset of diplopia (double vision). This is usually caused by a paresis of one of the extraocular muscles due to microvascular damage to the third, fourth, or the sixth cranial nerves [3,4].

When the extraocular muscle deficit is due to microvascular complications of diabetes the prognosis is good. Recovery of ocular motor function generally begins within three months of onset and recovery is usually complete. Although the diplopia can be debilitating, due to the generally limited course of these complaints, patients can usually be effectively managed conservatively with eye patching. When diplopia is from large divergence of the visual axes, patching one eye is the only practical short-term solution. When the deviation is smaller, the diplopia often can be resolved by using glasses with a horizontal or vertical prism or both. Surgery is rarely indicated.

If patients do not recover from a cranial nerve palsy within 6-12 months, eye muscle surgery to treat persistent and stable angle diplopia should be considered. These patients should consult with a neuro-ophthalmologist for continuing care.

3. Intraocular lens: Cataract

Cataract is a common cause of visual impairment in patients with diabetes. The Framingham study [5] revealed a three- to four fold increased prevalence of cataract in diabetic patients under the age of 65, and up to a twofold increased prevalence in patients above 65. Duration of diabetes and quality of glycemic control are the major risk factors for early cataract development [5].

Recurrent high levels of glucose in the lens lead to the glycolation of lens proteins from increased nonenzymatic glycation and oxidative stress to the lens [6]. This causes diabetic patients to develop age-related lens changes similar to nondiabetic age-related cataracts, except that they tend to occur at a younger age [7]. Several studies have analyzed the effect of vitamin and antioxidant supplements, such as vitamin C, E, and beta carotene and zinc, on preventing or slowing progression of age-related cataracts in diabetes without showing any statistically significant benefit with their use [6].

Early cataracts may cause mild visual impairment that can be managed reasonably with spectacle correction. Cataract surgery is indicated when visual function is significantly impaired by the cataract or if the cataract obscures the view of the retina and makes the diagnosis and treatment of diabetic retinopathy difficult.

Cataract surgery is safe in diabetic patients and there is a 95% success rate in terms of improved visual acuity [6]. Good glycemic control, fluid and electrolyte balance should be maintained perioperatively and the patient's treating physician and anesthesiologist should be involved in the process. It is recommended that the surgery be scheduled in the morning to minimize changes in the patient's usual schedule [8].

Some controversy exists regarding a potential association between cataract surgery and a subsequent worsening of diabetic retinopathy. Patients should be made aware of this risk preoperatively. Cataract surgery and its effect on diabetic retinopathy will be discussed in more detail in section 7.3.2.

4. Cornea

Corneal disorders secondary to diabetes (diabetic keratopathy) are increasingly recognized as a cause of ocular morbidity associated with diabetes. Patients with diabetes have structural changes of the corneal basement membrane that contributes to defects in the adhesion of corneal epithelial cells to the deeper stromal tissue [9]. This increases the risk of recurrent corneal erosions. In addition, accumulation of sorbitol in the cornea during periods of hyperglycemia leads to hypoesthesia (a loss of corneal sensation). Both hypoesthesia and epithelial adhesion dysfunction occur more frequently with increased severity and duration of diabetes. In patients with more long-standing or advanced diabetes, any corneal epithelial injury, either from trauma, during ocular surgery or from routine contact lens use, may result in prolonged healing times. This increases the risk of severe complications such as bacterial infiltration and ulceration.

Treatment of diabetic keratopathy is multifaceted, including artificial tears for mild cases, and the use of topical antibiotics, a bandage contact lens, eye patching, or closure for more severe cases.

5. Iris

Rubeosis iridis, neovascularization of the iris, is a serious complication of diabetes which occurs in patients with severe diabetic retinopathy [3]. Severe retinal ischemia stimulates the formation of numerous intertwining blood vessels on the anterior surface of the iris. These vessels can block aqueous outflow from the anterior chamber, leading to a sharp and persistent rise in intraocular pressure. This complication is known as neovascular glaucoma. This type of glaucoma is hard to treat and is often associated with pain from very high ocular pressure.

Topical medical therapy used commonly in other forms of glaucoma is less effective. Treatment should include aggressive control of the underlying diabetic retinopathy. The treatment of diabetic retinopathy will be discussed in more detail in section 7.

6. Retina – Diabetic retinopathy

Damage to the retinal capillaries, known as diabetic retinopathy, is the hallmark of diabetic eye disease. This condition is the major cause of blindness and visual disability in patients with type 1 diabetes.

There are two main pathways by which diabetic retinopathy can reduce vision: macular edema and proliferative retinopathy. These conditions can appear concomitantly or separately with the treatment protocol tailored to the relative severity each condition.

Macular edema develops when damaged retina vessels leak fluid and protein. These deposits collect on or under the macula of the eye where central vision is processed. This causes the macula to thicken and swell and may distort central vision.

Proliferative retinopathy occurs when diffuse injury to retinal vessels severely impairs retinal oxygenation. The hypoxia induces the release of proteins which stimulate the growth (or proliferation) of new, fragile retinal vessels. These new vessels have a propensity to bleed, which severely reduces vision.

In the following sections, we will discuss how retinopathy and macular edema develop and the various treatment options available to patients today, with a focus on exciting recent developments.

6.1. Epidemiology

Diabetic retinopathy is one of the most frequent causes of preventable blindness in working aged adults (20-74 years) [1,10]. In the USA, an estimated 86% of patients with type 1 diabetes have some degree of diabetic retinopathy. Data from the Wisconsin Epidemiologic Study of Diabetic Retinopathy (WESDR) showed that within 5 years of diagnosis of type 1 diabetes, 14% of patients developed retinopathy, with the incidence rising to 74% by 10 years [11,12]. In people with retinopathy at the WESDR baseline examination, 64% had their retinopathy worsen, 17% progressed to proliferative diabetic retinopathy (PDR), and about 20% developed diabetic macular edema during 10 years of follow-up.

The WESDR data in type 1 diabetics showed that 25 years after diagnosis, 97% of patients developed retinopathy, 43% progressed to PDR, 29% developed diabetic macular edema, and 3.6% of patients younger than 30 at diagnosis were legally blind [11]. The WESDR results also showed a reduction in the yearly incidence and progression of diabetic retinopathy during the past 15 years [12]. This may be signaling an improved ocular prognosis for diabetics today, possibly due to recent advances in glycemic control, ophthalmic treatment, and patient education.

The course of diabetic retinal disease in children with type 1 diabetes is fairly benign. Severe vision-reducing complications are uncommon in children before puberty [13].

6.2. Risk factors

There are several risk factors which influence the development and progression of diabetic retinopathy. The following list contains most of the important risk factors known today.

Modifiable risk factors:

1. **Hyperglycemia**: Good glycemic control has been shown to significantly prevent the development and progression of diabetic retinopathy. Every 1% decrease in hemoglobin A_{1C} leads to a 40% reduction in the risk of developing retinopathy, a 25% reduction in the risk of progression to vision-threatening retinopathy, and a 15% reduction in the risk of blindness [1,14,15].

2. **Hypertension**: Good blood pressure control is important in reducing the risk of retinopathy. Every 10 mmHg reduction in systolic blood pressure leads to a reduction of 35% in the risk of retinopathy progression and a reduction of 50% in the risk of visual loss [1].

3. **Obesity**: Obesity (BMI>30 kg/m(2)) is an important risk factor for diabetic retinopathy progression in type 1 diabetes, independent of HbA1c levels [16].

4. **Smoking**: There is some evidence that smoking may be a risk factor in progression of retinopathy in type 1 diabetes [17].

Nonmodifiable risk factors:

1. **Diabetes duration**: The longer the duration of diabetes, the higher the risk of developing diabetic retinopathy and of having a severe manifestation of this disease [1].

2. **Genetic factors**: The Diabetes Control and Complications Trial [18] showed a heritable tendency for developing diabetic retinopathy, regardless of other risk factors. The abnormal development of new blood vessels is regulated by protein called vascular endothelial growth factor A (VEGF –A). Variation in the sequence of this gene is associated with the development of severe diabetic retinopathy [19].

3. **Ethnicity**: Diabetic retinopathy in America is more prevalent among African Americans, Hispanic and south Asian groups than in Caucasians with otherwise similar risk profiles [1].

4. **Gender**: there is an observed gender dimorphism with younger females being at greater risk for diabetic retinopathy early in the course of diabetes [20] and males demonstrating greater risk later in life [21].

Other risk factors:

Pregnancy: Pregnancy is associated with worsening of diabetic retinopathy [22]. All pregnant women need to be closely monitored throughout pregnancy. Pregnancy in type 1 diabetes is discussed in further detail in section 7.3.1.

6.3. Pathophysiology

Diabetic retinopathy develops when hyperglycemia and other causal risk factors trigger a cascade of biochemical changes which damage retinal blood vessels. Hyperglycemia increases sorbitol levels via the action of aldose reductase increasing oxidative stress by reducing intracellular levels of reduced glutathione, an important antioxidant [23]. Intracellular hyperglycemia also increases synthesis of diacylglycerol, an activating cofactor for protein kinase C (PKC). Activated PKC decreases the production of anti-artherosclerotic factors and increases production of pro-artherogenic factors, pro-adhesive and pro-inflammatory factors [23]. As well, intracellular hyperglycemia leads to a rise in intracellular N-acetylglucosamine levels. This by-product reacts with serine and threonine residues in transcription factors, resulting in pathologic changes in gene expression [23]. The final by-product of these pathological processes is increased inflammation and increased oxidative stress, which causes endothelial cell dysfunction in retinal blood vessels.

Endothelial cell dysfunction induces retinal arteriolar dilatation, which increases capillary bed pressure. This results in microaneurysm formation, vessel leakage, and rupture [1]. Vascular permeability is also increased from loss of pericytes and increased endothelial proliferation in retinal capillaries. The breakdown of the blood–retinal barrier allows fluid to accumulate in the deep retinal layers where it damages photoreceptors and other neural tissues. This is the mechanism by which macular edema reduces visual acuity.

In some capillaries there is endothelial cell apoptosis. Vessels become acellular, leading to vascular occlusion and nonperfusion of local retinal tissue [23]. The resultant retinal ischemia promotes the release of inflammatory growth factors, such as vascular endothelial growth factor, growth-hormone-insulin growth factor, and erythropoietin [1]. These factors influence neovascularization, the growth of new capillaries, which are generally ineffective in improving tissue oxygenation as they often grow up toward the vitreous cavity.

6.4. Clinical features and classification

Diabetic retinopathy is classified as nonproliferative diabetic retinopathy (NPDR) when the vascular changes are limited to the retinal surface. It is classified as proliferative diabetic retinopathy (PDR) in the more advanced stage when new blood vessels form, which grow from the retinal surface up toward the vitreous cavity.

Diabetic macular edema occurs when leaky capillary beds allow fluid to accumulate in the part of the retina responsible for central vision. This complication can occur in patients with any level of underlying retinopathy from mild NPDR to severe PDR. Visual impairment is usually related to the state of macular disease and the consequences of neovascularization such as vitreous hemorrhage and retinal detachment. As such, the level of retinopathy does not always correlate with visual function, and severe diabetic retinopathy can be present initially without significant visual loss.

6.5. Diabetic macular edema

Diabetic macular edema (DME) is the complication of retinopathy responsible for most of the moderate visual loss in retinopathy patients. The loss of vision is often very mild at first, but without effective treatment it can progress and patients can lose the ability to perform activities of daily living such as reading and driving. Diabetic macular edema is assessed separately from the stage of retinopathy (NPDR/PDR) and it can manifest along a different and independent course.

The edema evolves when damage to the macular capillary bed causes increased retinal vascular permeability and fluid accumulation in the macula. Clinical examination can reveal rings of hard exudates (lipid-filled macrophages) that delineate the area of focal leakage.

Optical Coherence Tomography (OCT) is a useful ancillary imaging technique in DME. Recent technological advances in OCT technology have provided physicians with high-resolution images of the retina in cross-sectional slices. Aside from demonstrating areas of retinal thickening and intraretinal fluid, OCT obtains quantitative measurements of central retinal thickness. Serial OCT examinations are often used as a noninvasive and accurate method analyzing treatment response in DME patients [1].

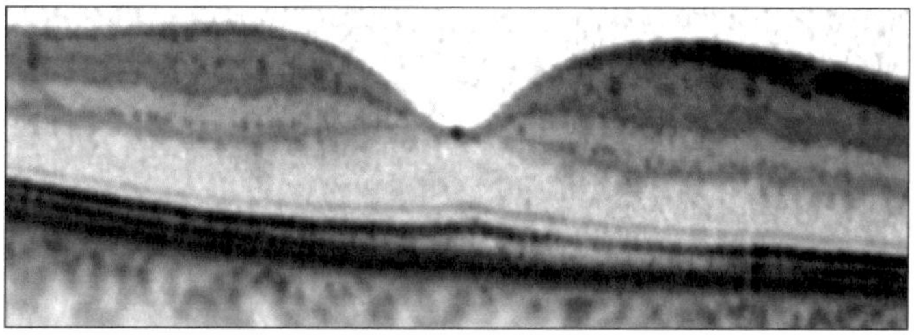

Figure 1. Normal OCT of the macular region.

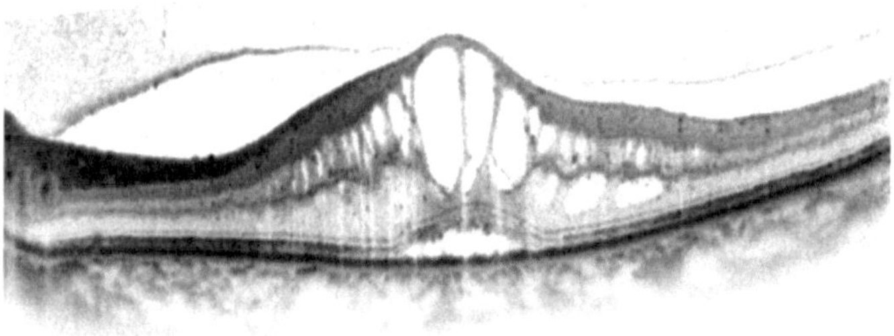

Figure 2. Macular edema: The OCT demonstrates the disruption of the normal macular anatomy due to macular edema.

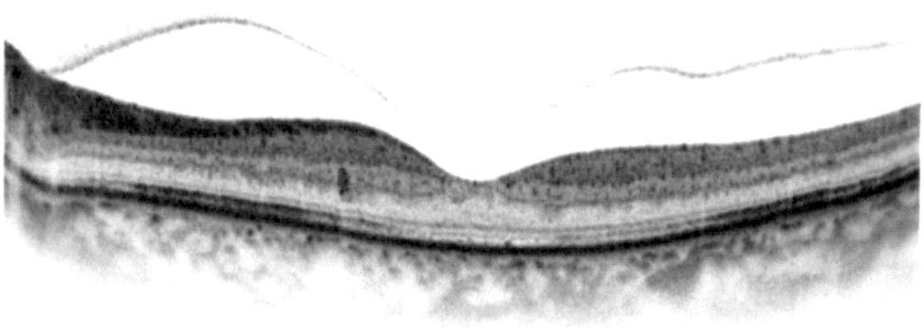

Figure 3. Posttreatment OCT: The same patient as in Figure 2 after treatment with intravitreal injections. The edema has been reabsorbed.

6.5.1. Nonproliferative Diabetic Retinopathy (NPDR)

In NPDR, the retinal microvascular changes do not extend beyond the surface of the retina. Clinical findings include microaneurysms (saccular enlargements of weakened capillaries), intraretinal hemorrhages, hard exudates (lipid-filled macrophages), cotton wool spots (nerve fiber layer infarcts), venous dilatations, and intraretinal microvascular abnormalities (dilated preexisting capillaries) [1,10].

NPDR is classified as mild, moderate, or severe, reflecting the risk of progression to PDR (Table 1) as determined by the Early Treatment in Diabetic Retinopathy Study [24].

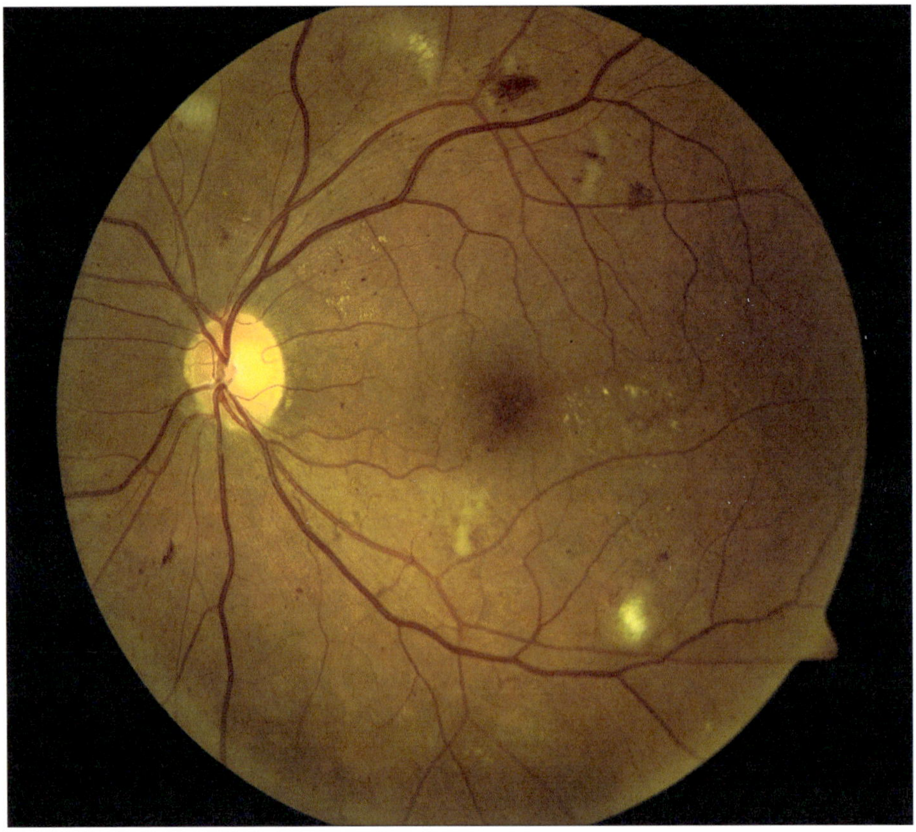

Figure 4. Nonproliferative diabetic retinopathy: Scattered hemorrhages ("dot and blot" shaped) can be seen throughout the retina.

6.5.2. Proliferative Diabetic Retinopathy (PDR)

Diabetic retinopathy advances to the proliferative stage when new vessels (neovascularizations) are formed which grow up from the retinal surface toward the vitreous cavity. The growth of these vessels is potentiated by the progression of diabetic retinal microvascular disease, causing severe retinal ischemia. This induces the release of proangiogenic factors

http://dx.doi.org/10.5772/61276

which promote the growth of these pathological vessels. Neovascularizations can be identified clinically as a jumble of disorganized, fine vessels emanating from the organized retinal vessel architecture. Angiography is also very effective at identifying neovascular lesions as the new vessels are porous and leak fluorescent dye into the vitreous cavity.

The new vessels in PDR evolve in three stages. Initially, the fine new vessels grow with minimal fibrous tissue. Then the new vessels increase in gauge and length with an increased fibrous component. Finally, the vessels regress and the residual fibrovascular tissue along the posterior surface of the vitreous body contracts.

Retinal neovascularizations (NV) are divided into two subtypes based on their relative risk of causing severe visual loss as demonstrated by the Diabetic Retinopathy Study (DRS). Vascular proliferations on or near the optic disc are termed NV-disc (NVD) and proliferations elsewhere are termed NV-elsewhere (NVE). The presence of NVD carries the higher risk of severe visual loss and requires more urgent treatment [25,26].

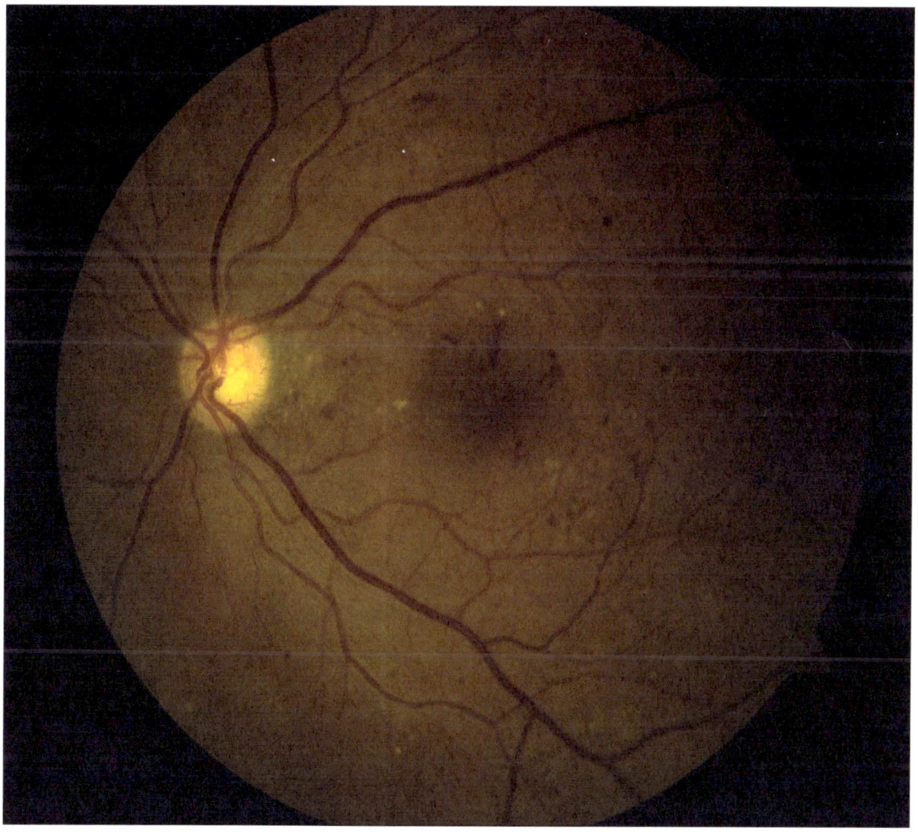

Figure 5. Neovascularization on the optic disc (NVD): The growth of fine new blood vessels can be seen on the optic disc. Urgent treatment is indicated to reduce the risk of vitreous hemorrhage.

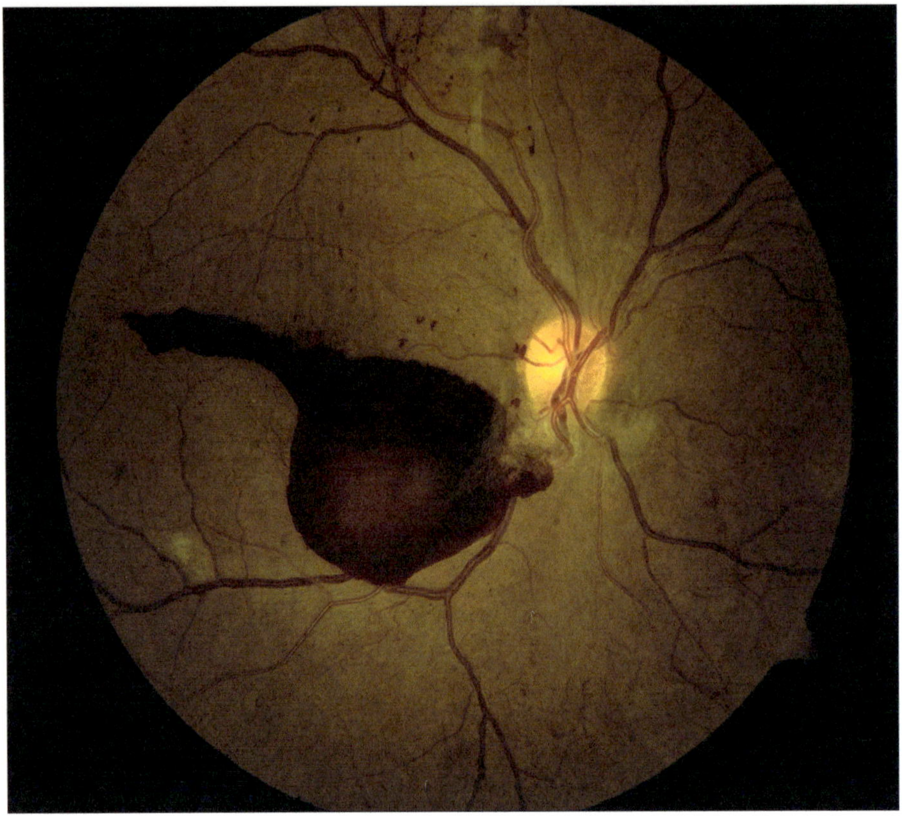

Figure 6. Vitreous hemorrhage with a neovascularization of the optic disc (NVD): The fragile blood vessels of the NVD have ruptured and a vitreous hemorrhage has collected, partially obscuring the macula and severely limiting vision.

PDR is graded from early to high risk according to the extent of the neovascular proliferations. The DRS [25,26] defined high-risk PDR as the presence of either: NVD with a vitreous hemorrhage, NVD larger than a quarter disc area without vitreous hemorrhage, or NVE larger than half disc area with vitreous hemorrhage. Without treatment, patients with early PDR have 50% risk of developing high-risk PDR in 1 year and those with high-risk PDR have a 25% risk of severe visual loss within 2 years. Treatment of PDR involving extensive peripheral laser ablation of the retina is discussed section 7.2.3.

The most common complication of PDR is vitreous hemorrhage caused by bleeding from the pathological neovascular vessels. Retinal detachments can also occur from the contraction of the neovascular tissue connecting the retinal surface to the vitreous.

Visual acuity in the absence of macular disease is often very good in PDR until a complication occurs; most commonly vitreous hemorrhage. This sudden transition from good vision to near blindness is often traumatic for patients who were unaware of the severity of their diabetic eye disease.

http://dx.doi.org/10.5772/61276

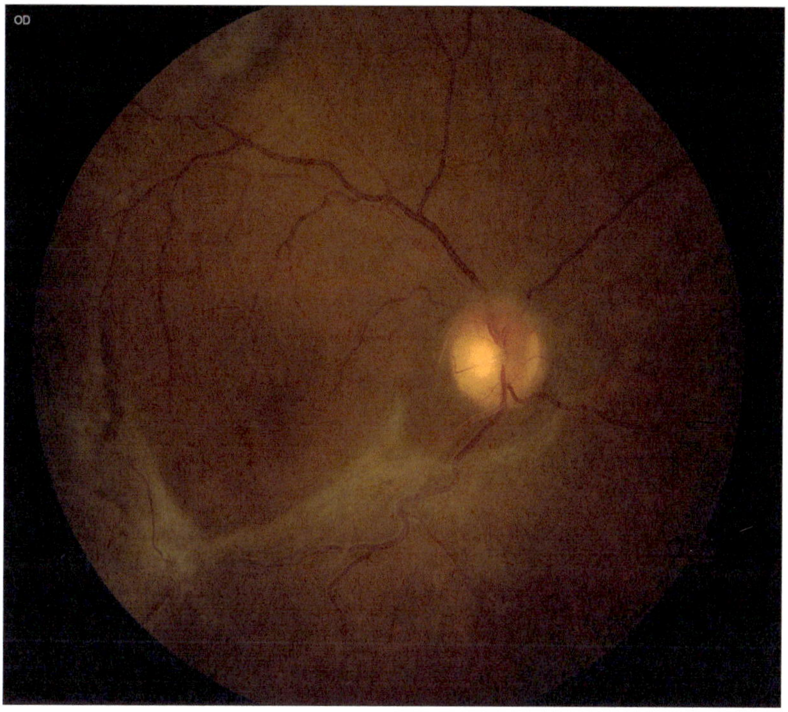

Figure 7. Traction Retinal Detachment: The neovascular tissue emanating from the optic disc and elsewhere has regressed leaving behind white fibrous tissue. This tissue has contracted and is distorting the retina in the macular region.

	Clinical Features	**Progression Risk**
Mild NPDR	Few microaneurysms	5% progress to PDR within 1 year
Moderate NPDR	Microaneurysms and other microvascular lesions	12-16% progress to PDR within 1 year
Severe NPDR (Meets 1 of 3 criteria)	• Extensive intraretinal hemorrhages and microaneurysms in all four quadrants • Venous beading in two or more quadrants • One IRMA	52% progress to PDR within 1 year 15% progress to high risk PDR within 1 year
Very severe NPDR	Any two of the features of severe NPDR	75% progress to PDR within 1 year 45% progress to high risk PDR within 1 year
Early PDR		50% risk of developing high risk PDR in 1 year
High risk PDR		25% risk of severe visual loss within 2 years

Table 1. Clinical classification of nonproliferative and proliferative diabetic retinopathy

7. Treatment of diabetic retinopathy

The main goal of treatment of diabetic retinopathy is to prevent complications that can lead to vision loss. Treatment should include both ocular therapy and systemic medical intervention.

7.1. Medical treatment

Hyperglycemia, hypertension, and hyperlipidemia are known risk factors for the development and progression of diabetic retinopathy. Treating and controlling these factors is crucial to preventing and limiting disease progression.

The Diabetes Control and Complications Trial [14] showed that intensive glycemic control reduced both the risk of developing retinopathy and the rate of progression of existing retinopathy. Intensive glycemic control reduced the risk for progression to severe NPDR and PDR, and the incidence of diabetic macular edema. Every percent reduction in hemoglobin A_{1C} lowers the risk of retinopathy development by 30-40%.

Antihypertensive treatment with ACE (angiotensin-converting enzyme) inhibitors can slow progression of diabetic nephropathy. The EUCLID study [27] investigated the effect of Lisinopril on progression of retinopathy in normotensive type 1 diabetics. They found that Lisinopril can decrease retinopathy progression in nonhypertensive patients who have type 1 diabetes with little or no nephropathy, although the mechanism is unclear. Unfortunately, other studies investigating the effect of ACE inhibitors on the progression of DR in type 1 diabetics have shown no significant benefits.

7.2. Ocular therapy

Ocular therapy in diabetic retinopathy includes panretinal or focal laser photocoagulation, intravitreal injections of either steroids or inhibitors of Vascular Endothelial Growth Factor (VEGF), surgery, or a combination of the aforementioned treatments. The suitable treatment regimen must be tailored individually for each patient and is based on clinical status of the patient (ocular and systemic), previous treatments, and data from the several reported and ongoing studies.

7.2.1. Diabetic macular edema treatment

Treatment options for diabetic macular edema (DME) include focal laser photocoagulation, intravitreal injections of either steroids or anti-VEGF compounds, and surgery.

7.2.1.1. Focal laser treatment

Until recently, the mainstay of DME treatment was macular laser photocoagulation. Treatment criteria are based on the ETDRS recommendations [24], which showed that eyes with macular edema involving or adjacent to the central macula, defined as clinically significant macular edema (CSME), benefited from macular laser treatment. Laser treatment reduced the risk of moderate visual loss (loss of three lines of vision) by 50% over 2 years compared with no treatment [24].

Macular laser treatment for CSME involves the application of discrete laser burns to areas of leakage in the macula. The treatment is not painful and can be repeated up to every 4 months.

Side effects of macular laser photocoagulation include: visual field loss, choroidal neovascularization, subretinal fibrosis, and inadvertent foveolar burns [10].

Modified photocoagulation techniques have been developed in response to these potential complications. The target of macular laser treatment for CSME is retinal pigment epithelium (RPE). Ideally, the laser energy would be absorbed only by the RPE and not spread to the surrounding tissues. Unfortunately, in conventional argon laser photocoagulation visible burns are created, indicating damage to the inner neural retina from the spread of thermal energy beyond the RPE.

Subthreshold diode laser micropulse (SDM) therapy delivers short pulses, which cause less thermal damage. Shorter laser exposure times confine the laser energy to a smaller zone, inflicting less damage on the neural retinal and choriocapillaries. SDM laser has been shown to be as effective as a conventional laser with fewer side effects [28].

7.2.1.2. Steroid injections

Inflammatory factors play an important role in the development of diabetic retinopathy. Upregulation of adhesion molecules in blood vessels leads to leukostasis and the accumulation of macrophages in the retinal vessels. These macrophages release angiogenic growth factors [29] and cytokines which increase vascular permeability. Glucocorticoids block the action of these macrophages and downregulate ICAM-1, which mediates leukocyte adhesion and transmigration [30].

In addition, glucocorticoids alter the composition of endothelial basal membrane by changing the local ratio of two laminin isoforms [31], suppressing basement membrane dissolution, and strengthening tight junctions to limit permeability and leakage that cause macular edema [32]. For this reason, it has long been thought that ocular steroid injections may be beneficial in DME treatment.

Intravitreal triamcinolone acetonide

Triamcinolone acetonide (TA) is a synthetic steroid of the glucocorticoid family with a molecular weight of 434.50. In 2001–2002, the first reports were published of the use of intravitreal injection of triamcinolone acetonide for DME [33,34]. The most common dose used is 4 mg.

Sutter et al. [35] reported in a prospective, double-masked, and randomized trial comparing 4 mg intravitreal TA with sham injection (saline). This study reported that 55% of 33 eyes treated with 4 mg of intravitreal TA improved by 5 or more letters of vision at 3 months compared with 16% of 32 eyes treated with sham injection.

The **DRCR.net** (diabetic retinopathy clinical research network) protocol I [36] studied the use of 4 mg TA combined with macular laser. It found that TA combined with laser significantly improved vision over macular laser alone in patients who had previously undergone cataract surgery. In patients who had not previously undergone cataract surgery TA was much less effective.

Potential side effects of corticosteroid injections include cataract formation and glaucoma. Moreover, as the treatment effect wanes, patients require repeated injections that increase the glaucoma and especially the cataract risk.

Instead of intermittent bolus therapy, it is thought that sustained release of a lower-dose glucocorticoid may lead to greater efficacy with fewer complications. This has led to the development of slow-release steroid implants.

Dexamethasone intravitreal implant

Dexamethasone is a strong synthetic member of the glucocorticoid class of steroid, with an anti-inflammatory and immunosuppressant activity 30 times greater than cortisol and 6 times greater than triamcinolone.

A sustained-release intravitreal dexamethasone (DEX) implant (Ozurdex®, Allergan Inc, Irvine, CA) is biodegradable and is placed in the vitreous cavity using a 22-gauge applicator through a small self-sealing puncture.

Dexmathasone implants have been examined in several large studies; The **PLACID** study [37] compared a DEX implant (0.7 mg) to treatment with focal laser. This 1-year study did not show a statistically significant visual improvement with the DEX implant.

The **MEAD** study [38] combined the results of two multicenter 3-year sham-controlled, masked, randomized clinical studies comparing DEX injection to focal laser treatment. Patients receiving the 0.7 DEX implant required mean of 4.1 injections over 3 years. The average visual improvement with the 0.7 mg DEX implant was +6 letters versus +1 letter with focal laser. Rates of cataract-related adverse events in phakic eyes were 67.9% and 20.4% in the DEX implant 0.7 mg, and sham groups, respectively. Two patients (0.6%) in the DEX implant 0.7 mg group required trabeculectomy for severe glaucoma. Based on the MEAD study, the Food and Drug Administration (FDA) approved DEX implants for use in DME.

Fluocinolone acetonide

Fluocinolone acetonide is a corticosteroid with average mass of 452 Da. ILUVIEN is a non-bioerodable intravitreal implant in a drug delivery system containing fluocinolone acetonide. The fluocinolone acetonide (FA) intravitreal implant [39] is administered in the clinic using a 25-gauge inserter designed to release the drug slowly over 36 months. Unlike the DEX implant, it is not bioerodable.

The FAME studies [40] were two phase 3 clinical trials examining the effect of long-acting fluocinolone acetonide inserts in patients with DME. Patients were randomized in a 2:2:1 ratio to the 0.2 μg per day FA implant, the 0.5 μg per day FA implant, or sham injection (saline). The mean improvement in BCVA letter score between baseline and month 24 was 4.4 and 5.4

in the low- and high-dose groups, respectively, compared with 1.7 in the sham group. Cataract extraction was performed 74.9% of all phakic subjects at baseline in the low-dose insert group and 84.5% in the high-dose insert group compared with 23.1% in the sham group.

Severely elevated intraocular pressure requiring glaucoma surgery occurred in 8.1% of patients in the high dose group, 5.8% of patients in the low dose group, compared only 0.5% in the sham treatment group [40].

This FA implant was approved in Europe (Austria, France, Germany, and Portugal) for the treatment of DME unresponsive to all other therapies. However, it was recently denied approval for this use by the US FDA, due to concerns centering on the high risk of severe glaucoma.

7.2.1.3. Anti-vascular endothelial growth hormone compounds

Vascular Endothelial Growth Hormone (VEGF) is a subfamily of growth factors produced by hypoxic cells that act as signal proteins to stimulate angiogenesis and vascular permeability. One of the main drivers of diabetic eye disease is damage to retinal blood vessels leading to tissue ischemia [41]. Hypoxic cells are then stimulated to release VEGF. Unsurprisingly, elevated levels of VEGF have been demonstrated in the eyes of patients with diabetic retinopathy [42,43]. Elevated VEGF stimulates both retinal vessel proliferation and increased vascular permeability producing the macular edema seen in diabetic eye disease [44].

The injection of anti-VEGF agents to the vitreous is both effective and safe. Adverse ocular effects with an incidence rate of less than 1% and include: cataract formation, retinal detachment, vitreous hemorrhage, and infection. Potential systemic adverse effects include: hypertension, stroke, and myocardial infarction but these are very uncommon [45]. Although there is a theoretical risk for arterial thromboembolic events in patients receiving VEGF-inhibitors by intravitreal injection, the observed incidence rate has been low in all studies and similar to that seen in patients randomized to placebo [1,46].

Over the past 10 years, anti-VEGF agents have become the first line of therapy in treating DME. There are three commercially available anti-VEGF agents: (i) Ranibizumab, (ii) Bevacizumab, and (iii) Aflibercept.

Ranibizumab

Ranibizumab (Lucentis®; Genentech, South San Francisco, California) is a humanized monoclonal antibody fragment directed at all isoforms of VEGF-A. Ranibizumab contains only the Fab fragment of the parental anti-VEGF antibody with weight of 48 kDa. Several large clinical trials have investigated the role of Ranibizumab in the treatment of diabetic macular edema.

READ-2 [47] was a 6-month multicenter trial where patients were randomized in a 1:1:1 fashion to macular laser; monthly Ranibizumab; or a combination of laser and monthly Ranibizumab. At 6 months, the combination therapy and Ranibizumab-only groups gained 3.80 and 7.2 letters at month 6, respectively, compared with no change in the laser only group.

RESTORE [48] was a similar 12-month phase 3 clinical trial which compared Ranibizumab to both laser alone and to laser combined with Ranibizumab. All patients receiving Ranibizumab received three initial consecutive monthly injections followed by pro re nata (PRN, as needed) injections as determined at the monthly examination. At month 12, both the Ranibizumab alone and Ranibizumab with laser groups improved by 6 letters, while the laser alone group remained nearly unchanged. Patients required a mean of seven Ranibizumab injections and the change in vision was statistically significant.

As the data supporting Ranibizumab supplanting laser for primary treatment of center-involving DME grew, many physicians were unsure of the continuing role of focal laser in DME. To answer this among other questions, the **DRCR.net** [49,50] performed a randomized trial which notably compared two methods of combining adjuvant laser with Ranibizumab injections. In one arm of the study (prompt laser), focal laser was given to all the patients at initiation and repeated every 4 months as needed. In the other arm (delayed laser), focal laser could only be added if the edema persisted beyond 24 weeks of monthly Ranibizumab treatment. After 3 years of follow-up, the average gain in the prompt laser group was 7 letters compared with 10 letters in the delayed laser group. Based on these results, it is generally accepted that treatment for center-involving DME should begin with an anti-VEGF agent. Focal laser may be added only if the edema is persistent despite several consecutive anti-VEGF injections. The FDA approved Ranibizumab for treatment of DME in 2012.

Bevacizumab

Bevacizumab (Avastin®; Genentech, South San Francisco, California) is a full-length recombinant humanized monoclonal immunoglobulin G1κ antibody weighing 149 kDa which inactivates all VEGF isoforms. It was FDA-approved in 2004 as a treatment for colon cancer. However, as emerging evidence pointed to VEGF as a central player in DME, ophthalmologists began to use bevacizumab as an "off-label" treatment.

One of the criticisms of Bevacizumab use is that it has not been specifically formulated for ocular use. Bevacizumab is sold in large vials intended for intravenous uses and compounding pharmacies aliquot the medication into prefilled syringes for ocular use. Although there have been case reports of contamination due to this extra step in the preparation process, the safety of Bevacizumab for ocular use has been well established in trials for Age-related Macular Degeneration with a side-effect profile similar to Ranibizumab [51].

Bevacizumab has yet to be approved by the FDA for use in DME. Despite this it is used in many jurisdictions because of its efficacy and its significantly lower cost compared with Ranibizumab. One study [52] estimated the cost of treating DME with Ranibizumab was 20-fold higher than treating with Bevacizumab.

BOLT [53], a 2-year trial comparing bevacizumab monotherapy with focal laser, is the best randomized trial supporting the use of Bevacizumab for center-involving DME. Eighty patients with center-involved DME were randomized to receive either every 6-weekly intravitreal bevacizumab injections (1.25 mg) or focal laser monotherapy.

At 2 years, there was a mean gain of 8.6 letters for Bevacizumab alone compared with a mean loss of 0.5 letters in the laser group.

Aflibercept

Aflibercept (EYLEA®-Regeneron Pharmaceuticals, Tarrytown, New York, NY, and Bayer Healthcare Pharmaceuticals, Berlin, Germany) is a 115-kDa anti-VEGF agent. This protein was developed by combining the extracellular binding domains of VEGF receptors1 and 2 to the Fc segment of human immunoglobulin-G1.Similar to Ranibizumab and Bevacizumab, Aflibercept binds to all isomers of the VEGF-A family.

The phase II **DA VINCI** [54] trial compared two doses of Aflibercept, 0.5 mg and 2.0 mg, to laser treatment. The average improvement in visual acuity at 52 weeks was +11 letters for monthly 0.5 mg, +13 letters for monthly 2.0 mg and −1 letters for laser alone.

A separate arm of this trial received 3 monthly 2 mg doses followed by a scheduled dose every 8 weeks. Patients in this arm received an average of 7.2 injections per year, as compared with over 12 for monthly dosing. The average visual change was +10 letters. Ocular adverse events were consistent with those seen in other trials with anti-VEGF drugs.

The recently completed phase III **VIVID** [55] and **VISTA** [56] trials were similarly designed. Both supported the finding that a schedule of 5 monthly doses of Aflibercept followed by regular bimonthly dosing was of similar efficacy to continuous monthly injections.

In 2014, FDA approved EYLEA for the treatment of diabetic macular edema. The recommended dosage is 2 mg every 2 months, after five initial monthly injections.

Method of administration

The injection procedure should be carried out under aseptic conditions, which includes the use of surgical hand disinfection, sterile gloves, a sterile drape, and a sterile eyelid speculum (or equivalent). Adequate anaesthesia and a broad-spectrum topical microbicide to disinfect the periocular skin, eyelid and ocular surface should be administered prior to the injection, in accordance with local practice.

The injection needle should be inserted 3.5-4.0 mm posterior to the limbus into the vitreous cavity, avoiding the horizontal meridian and aiming toward the center of the globe. The injection volume of 0.05 ml is then delivered.

The use of pre- or postinjection topical antibiotics is not recommended as they have not been shown to alter the infection risk [57].

7.2.2. Nonproliferative diabetic retinopathy treatment

Visual acuity is not usually affected in nonproliferative diabetic retinopathy unless there is damage to the macula in the form of macular edema or ischemia. Ocular treatment at this stage is definitively indicated only if there is evidence of macular disease.

7.2.3. Proliferative diabetic retinopathy treatment

The goal of treatment in proliferative diabetic retinopathy (PDR) is to prevent complications and lower the risk of severe vision loss. The mainstay of treatment for PDR is laser ablation of the peripheral retina where laser burns are placed over the entire retina, sparing the central macula. This treatment is called panretinal photocoagulation (PRP). PRP promotes the regression and arrest of progression of retinal neovascularizations by destroying ischemic retinal tissue and reducing ischemia-driven VEGF production [1,10].

The Diabetic Retinopathy Study (DRS) [25,26] evaluated efficacy of PRP treatment in eyes with advanced NPDR or PDR (DRS Group, 1981). The **DRS** study recommended prompt treatment in eyes with high-risk PDR (defined in section 6.4.3), because these eyes had the highest risk for severe visual loss. PRP treatment in these patients reduced the risk of severe visual loss by 50% over 5 years.

The **ETDRS** study [24,58] found that PRP treatment in eyes with early PDR reduced the risk of progression to high-risk PDR by 50%, and significantly reduced the risk of severe visual loss [24]. Based on these results, PRP treatment should be considered in eyes with any stage PDR especially if there is poor metabolic control, a noncompliant patient, or difficulty in maintaining close follow-up.

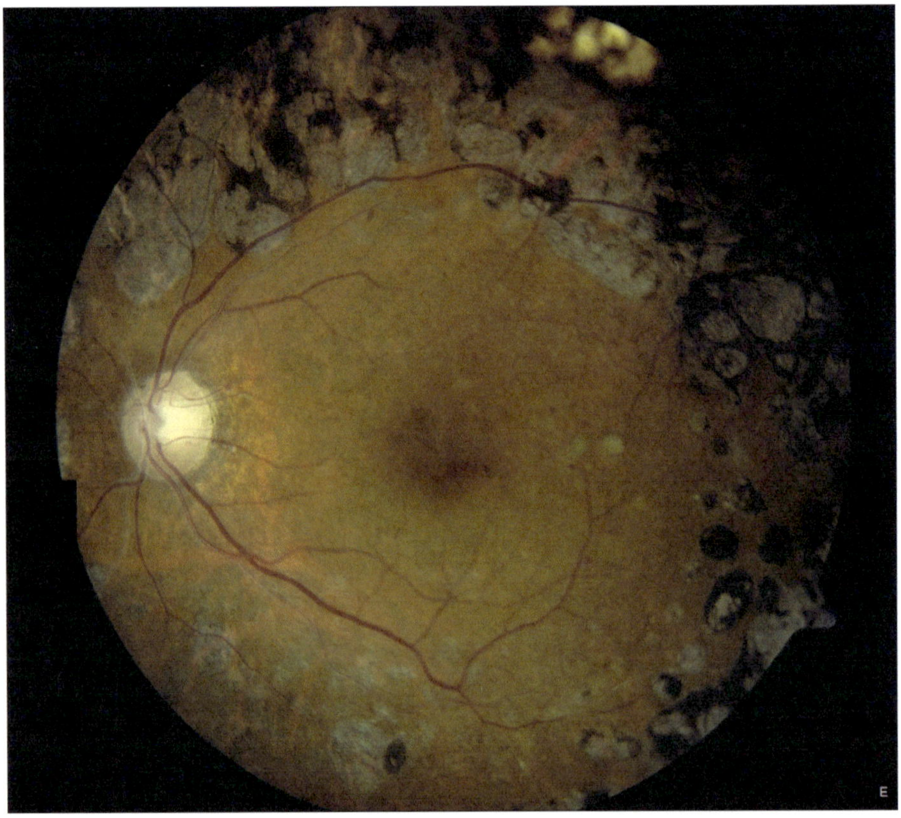

Figure 8. Panretinal photocoagulation: The retinal tissue surrounding the macular region has been ablated using Argon laser. Circular grey-black scars demark areas previously treated with laser burns.

Full PRP treatment as recommended by the **DRS** [25,26] and the **ETDRS** [24,58] includes as many as 5000 laser burns. PRP can be painful and is often performed over several sessions. After the initial treatment course, additional therapy can be applied if there is persistent neovascularization. After treatment, proliferative retinal tissue may regress and contract causing a vitreous hemorrhage or a traction retinal detachment from contracture of fibrovascular tissue. Side effects of PRP treatment also include decreased in night vision, decreased color vision, and loss of peripheral vision [10].

When PDR presents with macular edema, PRP treatment may initially increase the amount of edema [58]. In such case, it is recommended to treat the macular edema with an intravitreal injection before initiating PRP [59,60].

7.2.3.1. *Surgery in proliferative diabetic retinopathy*

Vitrectomy surgery is most commonly performed in PDR for a dense vitreous hemorrhage causing severe vision loss. If an eye which has not previously undergone PRP develops a significant hemorrhage and vision loss, vitrectomy is recommended when the hemorrhage persists beyond 1–3 months. Patients with vitreous hemorrhage that have preexisting complete PRP may undergo a longer observation period as many patients will have a spontaneous improvement beyond the initial 4 weeks [10,61]. Traction retinal detachment induced by the contraction of neovascular tissue connecting the retinal surface to the vitreous is another serious complication of PDR. If central vision is affected surgery is recommended. However, traction detachments which do not involve the central macula can remain stable for years. Surgery is indicated only when the traction retinal detachment involves or threatens the central macula or if a retinal tear develops [10].

Common complications after vitrectomy include corneal epithelial defects, cataract formation, elevated intraocular pressure, recurrent vitreous hemorrhage, iatrogenic retinal breaks, and rhegmatogenous retinal detachment. The development of these complications can be minimized by meticulous surgical technique and cautious postoperative follow-up.

7.2.3.2. *Role of anti-VEGF agents*

Several studies have evaluated the efficacy of adjunctive intravitreal anti-VEGF injections in patients with PDR [46]. Adding an anti-VEGF agent to eyes undergoing PRP reduces the risk of a vitreous hemorrhage 12 months after PRP [62]. In eyes with PDR and a dense vitreous hemorrhage, a Bevacizumab injection has been shown to aid significantly in clearing the hemorrhage [63]. This allows PRP to be completed and may reduce the number of patients ending up in surgery.

Bevacizumab has also been shown to enhance retinal surgery in patients with PDR. A single Bevacizumab injection given 1 week before vitrectomy for vitreous hemorrhage, results in decreased bleeding during surgery, decreased operating time, and less postoperative vitreous hemorrhage as compared to vitrectomy [46,64]. As separate study found that a preoperative Bevacizumab injection improved visual acuity 12 months postoperatively compared with vitrectomy alone [62].

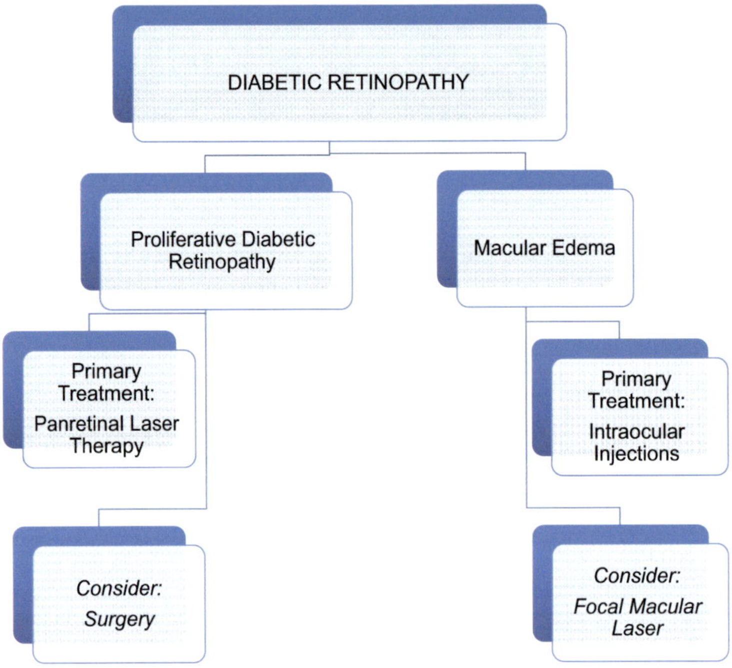

Figure 9. Summary of the two main pathways by which diabetic retinopathy can reduce vision.

7.3. Special considerations

7.3.1. Diabetic retinopathy in pregnancy

In women with preexisting diabetes, pregnancy is considered an independent risk factor for the development and progression of diabetic retinopathy [65]. Most of the progression of diabetic retinopathy in pregnancy occurs by the end of the second trimester. Although regression of retinopathy usually occurs postpartum, there is still an increased risk for progression during the first year postpartum [65]. Risk factors for the development and progression of diabetic retinopathy in pregnancy include longer duration of diabetes before conception, rapid normalization of hemoglobin $A1_C$ at the beginning of pregnancy, poor glycemic control during pregnancy, diabetic nephropathy, high blood pressure, and preeclampsia [65,66].

Severity of diabetic retinopathy before or at beginning of pregnancy is also a strong predictor of progression of retinopathy during and after pregnancy. The **Diabetes in Early Pregnancy Study** [67] showed that 10.3% of women without diabetic retinopathy and 18.8% with mild NPDR experienced retinopathy progression during pregnancy, and 6.3% of women with mild NPDR progressed to PDR. In women with moderate NPDR, 54.8% suffered retinopathy progression and 29% developed PDR. Overall, progression to sight-threatening diabetic retinopathy, including macular edema and PDR, occurs in 6% of pregnant diabetic women [66].

Progression of retinopathy during pregnancy is probably related to the hypervolemic and hypercoagulable states in pregnancy, as well as elevated pro-inflammatory and angiogenic factor levels. This results in capillary occlusion and leakage-aggravating diabetic retinopathy mechanisms [65,68]. Ideally, good glycemic control and full treatment of preexisting diabetic retinopathy complications should be attained before conception.

All diabetic women who plan pregnancy should be referred by their treating physician to an ophthalmologist. The recommended follow-up of pregnant women with type 1 diabetes includes an ophthalmologic exam at the beginning of pregnancy and during the first trimester. Subsequent follow-up depends on the stage of diabetic retinopathy found on the initial examinations. In women with no retinopathy or very mild NPDR, an ophthalmologic exam is indicated when there are visual complaints. In moderate NPDR, an exam should be done at least once during the second trimester and every 4–6 weeks during the third trimester. In severe NPDR and PDR, close follow-up is needed, and an exam should be done every 4–6 weeks, from the beginning of the second trimester.

Treatment of diabetic retinopathy during pregnancy includes maximal control of both glucose levels and blood pressure [66]. Ocular therapy such as PRP should definitely be performed for PDR and be strongly considered in cases of severe NPDR. Disease progression can be very fast in pregnancy and waiting for PDR to clearly develop may result in severe complications that necessitate invasive surgery. Ocular therapy for PDR and macular edema during pregnancy can include PRP, focal laser, and intravitreal steroid injections. Although there are not much data on the safety of intravitreal injections of anti-VEGF agents during pregnancy, the literature includes some reports on the safe and effective use of Bevacizumab [69].

7.3.2. Cataract surgery in patients with diabetic retinopathy

Cataract development is major factor compromising vision in diabetic patients. Surgery often results in significant vision improvements but these can be mitigated by the progression of diabetic retinopathy and macular edema.

7.3.2.1. Macular edema progression following cataract extraction

Progression of macular edema following cataract extraction can limit the expected improvement in visual acuity from cataract surgery. The reported rates of macular edema following cataract extraction varies from 4% to 70%, depending upon the method used to identify macular edema (angiographic, biomicroscopic, OCT), the cataract extraction technique, and underlying comorbidities [70,71].

The **DRCR.net** [72] conducted a multicenter, prospective, observational study including 293 participants with diabetic retinopathy but without significant macular edema requiring treatment. The authors concluded that in eyes with diabetic retinopathy, the presence of noncentral-involved macular edema immediately prior to cataract surgery, or a history of macular edema treatment may increase the risk of developing central-involving macular edema 16 weeks after cataract extraction.

Topical Nonsteroidal Anti-inflammatory Agents

Controlling postsurgical inflammation is an important factor in preventing macular edema development. Prostaglandin release considerably contributes to fluid leakage from perifoveal capillaries into the extracellular space of the macular region. Multiple studies have reported the benefits of using nonsteroidal anti-inflammatory eye drops pre- and postoperatively to reduce the rate of edema progression [73,74].

Antivascular Endothelial Growth Factor Injections

Recent studies have shown a potential benefit using intravitreal anti-VEGF injections at the end of cataract surgery especially in cases with poorly controlled or refractory macular edema before surgery [46,75,76]. High-risk patients who received intravitreal Bevacizumab or Ranibizumab benefit from better outcomes in terms of visual acuity, macular thickness, and retinopathy progression.

7.3.2.2. Diabetic retinopathy progression following cataract extraction

Controversy exists in the ophthalmic community as to whether cataract surgery potentiates diabetic retinopathy progression. Several studies have reported worsening of diabetic retinopathy and macular edema after surgery [77-80]. Progression was seen during the first year after surgery and was highest in the first 3 months postoperatively. A review of several other studies, especially in the era of cataract surgery using the smaller incision phacoemulsification technique, showed no significant progression of diabetic retinopathy and macular edema after surgery [81,82]. Overall, it is likely that uncomplicated phacoemulsification does not result in a substantially increased risk of the DR progression [83]. The observed rates of progression after uncomplicated, small-incision surgery are similar to the natural course of retinopathy progression over time. The vision improvement and the ability to better visualize the retina to monitor retinopathy progression clearly outweigh the current risks of modern-day cataract extraction and subsequent retinopathy progression over time [83], Overall, diabetics with cataracts benefit from surgery, and improved visual acuity is reported in 92–94% of patients [81]. The combined evidence suggests that in patients with low risk or absent diabetic retinopathy, there is no increased risk of retinopathy progression. However, patients with more advanced retinopathy have an increased risk for retinopathy progression and a worse visual acuity outcome.

7.3.2.3. Summary

A thorough evaluation of patients with diabetes is warranted before cataract surgery. Patients who have severe NPDR or PDR should be considered for PRP treatment prior to cataract removal [84]. Patients with significant macular edema should undergo treatment with a steroid or anti-VEGF agent preoperatively. Ideally, surgery should be delayed until stabilization of retinopathy and macular edema is achieved. In refractory cases, adjunctive therapy with a steroid of anti-VEGF agent at the end of cataract surgery should be considered. Close postoperative follow-up with an ophthalmologist is highly recommended in all patients with preexisting diabetic retinopathy.

8. Schedule for ophthalmologic examinations

Regular ocular examination can detect early ocular disease such as cataracts and glaucoma as well as retinopathy. Diabetic retinopathy in type 1 diabetes is rare during the first 5 years after diagnosis, so the baseline ophthalmologic examination could be extended to 5 years after diagnosis. In children with prepubertal diabetes, the baseline examination should be done at puberty [13].

The timing and frequency of follow-up ocular examinations depends on individual patient's status. In high-risk patients with long-term diabetes and poor systemic risk factor control, annual examinations should be performed even in the absence of retinopathy. In patients with known retinopathy, the examination schedule is based on the degree of retinopathy, and on the patient's compliance and adherence to regular follow-up. In mild NPDR, an examination should be performed every 9–12 months; in moderate NPDR, every 6 months; and in severe NPDR, PDR and CSME follow-up should be even more frequent even in the absence of ongoing treatment [10].

Severity ofRetinopathy	Follow-up Schedule (Months)
None or minimal NPDR	12
Mild NPDR	9-12
Moderate NPDR	6
Severe NPDR	2-4
Non-high-risk PDR	2-4
High-risk PDR	2-4
Diabetic macular edema	1-3

NPDR = non-proliferative diabetic retinopathy; PDR = proliferative diabetic retinopathy

Table 2. Diabetic retinopathy (follow-up recommendations)

9. Conclusion

Diabetes is the leading cause of vision loss in working-age patients, mainly due to diabetic retinopathy. The mainstay in the prevention of disease progression remains optimizing glycemic control and controlling other ancillary risk factors. Laser treatments which prevent vision loss remain an important option for many patients with advanced diabetic retinopathy. Recent advances in medical treatment over the past decade, especially intraocular injections for macular edema, show great promise due to their ability to improve vision. Today, more than ever before, patients with even advanced diabetic eye disease have a good chance of maintaining functional vision for many years provided they undergo proper screening to diagnose complications as they arise. The cost of these new treatments is significant both in financial terms and in terms of patient time investment, as frequent, often monthly, clinic visits are often recommended to optimize results. Additional studies are still needed in order to develop more effective and less costly treatments to further improve the visual prognosis for diabetic patients.

Author details

Efraim Berco[1,2], Daniel Rappoport[1,2], Ayala Pollack[1,2], Guy Kleinmann[1,2] and Yoel Greenwald[1,2]*

*Address all correspondence to: yoel.greenwald@gmail.com

1 Ophthalmology Department, Kaplan Medical Center, Rehovot, Israel

2 Hebrew University and Hadassah Medical School, Jerusalem, Israel

References

[1] Cheung N, Mitchell P,Wong TY. Diabetic Retinopathy. *The Lancet* 2010; 376: 124-36. DOI: 10.1016/S0140-6736(09)62124-3.

[2] Fauci AS, Brownwald E, Kasper DL et al. (Eds.) McGraw-Hill Powers AC. Diabetes Mellitus. *Harrison's Principles of Internal Medicine*. Retrieved from: http://www.accessmedicine.com

[3] Thomas D, Graham E. Ocular disorders associated with systemic disease. In: Riordan-Eva P & Whitcher JP (Eds.) *Vaughan & Asbury's General Ophthalmology*, McGraw-Hill,2008. Retrieved from: http://www.accessmedicine.com

[4] Kline LB, Tariq-Bhatti M, Chung SM et al. (Eds.) Section 5: Neuro-ophthalmology. *Basic and Clinical Science Course, -2011,American Academy of Ophthalmology*. American Academy of Ophthalmology.

[5] Leibowitz HM, Krueger DE, Dawber TR et al. The Framingham Eye Study monograph: An ophthalmological and epidemiological study of cataract, glaucoma, diabetic retinopathy, macular degeneration, and visual acuity in a general population of 2631 adults, 1973-1975. *Surv Ophthalmol* 1980; 24:335-610

[6] Obrosova SS, Chung SS, Kador PF. Diabetic cataracts: mechanisms and management. *Diabetes/Metabol Res Rev* 2010:26(3):172-180. DOI:10.1002/dmrr. 1075

[7] Bobrow JC, Blecher MH, Glasser D et al. (Eds.). Section 11: Lens and cataract. *Basic and Clinical Science Course, 2010-2011, American Academy of Ophthalmology.* Americam Academy of Ophthalmology.

[8] Purdy EP, Bolling JP, Di-Lorenzo AL et al. (Eds.) Endocrine disorders. In: Section 1: Update on general medicine. *Basic and Clinical Science Course 2010-2011, American Academy of Ophthalmology. 2010;* 189-205, American Academy of Ophthalmology.

[9] Reidy JJ, Bouchard CS, Florakis GJ et al. (Eds.) Metabolic disorders with corneal changes. In: Section 8: External disease and cornea. *Basic and Clinical Science Course 2010-2011, American Academy of Ophthalmology. 2010;* 307-308. American Academy of Ophthalmology.

[10] Regillo C, Holekamp N, Johnson MW et al. (Eds.) Retinal vascular disease: Diabetic retinopathy. Section 12, Retina and vitreous. *Basic and Clinical Science Course, 2010-2011, American Academy of Ophthalmology.* 2010;109-132. American Academy of Ophthalmology.

[11] Klein R, Knudtson MD, Lee KF et al. The Wisconsin Epidemiologic Study of Diabetic Retinopathy: XXII the twenty-five-year progression of retinopathy in persons with type 1 diabetes. *Ophthalmology* 2008;115(11):1859-1868. doi: 10.1016/j.ophtha. 2008.08.023.

[12] Varma R. From a population to patients: The Wisconsin Epidemiologic Study of Diabetic Retinopathy. *Ophthalmology* 2008; 115(11):1857-1858. DOI: 10.1016/j. ophtha. 2008.09.023.

[13] Raab EL, Aaby AA, Bloom JN et al. (Eds.) Vitreous and retinal diseases and disorders. In: Section 6: Pediatric ophthalmology and strabismus. *Basic and Clinical Science Course 2010-2011, American Academy of Ophthalmology. 2010;* 296-297/ American Academy of Ophthalmology.

[14] DCCT 1995: Progression of retinopathy with intensive versus conventional treatment in the Diabetes Control and Complications Trial. Diabetes Control and Complications Trial Research Group. *Ophthalmology* 1995;102(4): 647-661.

[15] Scanlon PH, Aldington SJ, Stratton IM. Epidemiological issues in diabetic retinopathy. *Middle East Afr J Ophthalmol* 2014;20:293-300. DOI: 10.4103/0974-9233.120007

[16] Price SA, Gorelik A, Wentworth JM et al. Obesity is associated with retinopathy and macrovascular disease in type 1 diabetes. *Obes Res Clin Pract* 2014;8:178-182. DOI: 10.1016/j.orcp.2013.03.007.

[17] Karamanos B, Porta M, Fuller JH et al. Different risk factors of microangionpathy in patients with type 1 diabetes mellitus of short versus long duration. The EURODIAB IDDM complications study. *Diabetologia*. 2000;43:348-355.

[18] DCCT 1997: Clustering of long term complications in families with diabetes in the diabetes control and complications trial. The Diabetes Control and Complications Trial Research Group. *Diabetes* 1997;46(11):1829-1839.

[19] Han L, Zhang L, Zhao J et al. The associations between VEGF gene polymorphisms and diabetic retinopathy susceptibility: a meta-analysis of 11 case-control studies. *J Diabetes Res* 2014;2014 DOI:10.1155/2014/805801.

[20] Gallego PH, Craig ME, Donaghue KC et al. Role of blood pressure in development of early retinopathy in adolescents with type 1 diabetes: Prospective cohort study. *BMJ* 2008;337: 918. DOI: 10.1136/bmj.a918.

[21] Harjutsalo V, Maric C, Groop PH, Finn Diane Study Group. Sex-related differences in the long-term risk of microvascular complications by age at onset of type 1 diabetes. *Diabetologia* 2011;54:1992-1999. DOI: 10.1007/s00125-011-2144-2

[22] DCCT 2000: Effect of pregnancy on microvascular complications in the diabetes control and complications trial. The Diabetes Control and Complications Trail Research Group. *Diabetes Care* 2000; 23(8):1084-1091.

[23] Stirban A, Rosen P, Tschoepe D. Complications of type 1 diabetes: new molecular findings. *Mount Sinai J Med* 2008; 75(4): 328-351. DOI: 10/1002/msj. 20057.

[24] ETDRS 1995: Focal photocoagulation treatment of diabetic macular edema: relationship of treatment effect to fluorescein angiographic and other retinal characteristics at baseline. ETDRS Report 19. Early Treatment Diabetic Retinopathy Study Research Group. *Arch Ophthalmol* 1995;113(9):1144-1155.

[25] DRS 1979: Four risk factors for severe visual loss in diabetic retinopathy. DRS Report 3. Diabetic Retinopathy Study Research Group. *Arch Ophthalmol* 1979; 97(4): 654-655.

[26] DRS 1981: Photocoagulation treatment of proliferative diabetic retinopathy: clinical application of Diabetic Retinopathy Study (DRS) findings. DRS Report 8. Diabetic Retinopathy Study Research Group. *Ophthalmology* 1981;88(7):583-600.

[27] Chaturvedi N, Fuller JH, Aiello LP, EUCLID study Group. Circulating plasma vascular endothelial growth factor and microvascular complications of type 1 diabetes mellitus: the influence of ACE inhibition. *Diabet Med.* 2001;18:288-294.

[28] Venkatesh P, Ramanjulu R, Garg S et al. Subthreshold micropulse diode laser and double frequency neodymium: YAG laser in treatment of diabetic macular edema: a prospective, randomized study using multifocal electroretinography. *Photomed Laser Surg* 2011;29:727-733. DOI: 10.1089/pho.2010.2830.

[29] Ingber DE, Madri JA, Folkman J. A possible mechanism for inhibition of angiogenesis by angiostatic steroids: induction of capillary basement membrane dissolution. *Endocrinology*1986;119(4):1768-1775.

[30] Stokes CL, Weisz PB, Williams SK et al. Inhibition of microvascular endothelial cell migration by beta-cyclodextrin tetradecasulfate and hydrocortisone. *Microvas Res* 1990;40(2):279-284.

[31] Tokida Y, Aratani Y, Morita A et al. Production of two variant laminin forms by endothelial cells and shift of their relative levels by angiostatic steroids. *J Biol Chem* 1990;265(30):18123-9.

[32] Ciulla TA, Harris A, McIntyre N, Jonescu-Cuypers C. Treatment of diabetic macular edema with sustained-release glucocorticoids: intravitreal triamcinolone acetonide, dexamethasone implant, and fluocinolone acetonide implant. *Rev Expert Opin Pharmacother* 2014;15:953-959. DOI: 10.1517/14656566.2014.896899

[33] Jonas JB, Söfker A. Intraocular injection of crystalline cortisone as adjunctive treatment of diabetic macular edema. *Am J Ophthalmol* 2001;132:425-427.

[34] Martidis A, Duker JS, Baumal C et al. Intravitreal triamcinolone for refractory diabetic macular edema. *Ophthalmology* 2002;109:920-927.

[35] Sutter FK, Simpson JM, Gillies MC et al. Intravitreal triamcinolone for diabetic macular edema that persists after laser treatment: three-month efficacy and safety results of a prospective, randomized, double-masked, placebo-controlled clinical trial. *Ophthalmology* 2004;111:2044-2049.

[36] DRCR network 2010a: The Diabetic Retinopathy Clinical Research Network. Randomized trial evaluating Ranibizumab plus prompt or deferred laser or Triamcinolone plus prompt laser for diabetic macular edema. *Ophthalmology* 2010;117(6): 1067-1077. DOI: 10.1016/j.ophtha.2010.02.031.

[37] Callanan D, Gupta S, Boyer D et al. Dexamethasone intravitreal implant in combination with laser photocoagulation for the treatment of diffuse diabetic macular edema. *Ophthalmology* 2013;120;1843-1851. DOI: 10.1016/j.ophtha.2013.02.018

[38] Sadda S, Boyer D, He Yoon Y et al. Safety and efficacy of dexamethasone intravitreal implant in patient with diabetic macular edema: phase III, 3 year, randomized, sham-controlled study [MEAD]. 2014;10:1904-1914. DOI: 10.1016/j.ophtha.2014.04.024

[39] Campochiaro PA, Hafiz G, Shah SM et al. Famous Study Group. Sustained ocular delivery of fluocinolone acetonide by an intravitreal insert. *Ophthalmology* 2010;117(7): 1393-1399. DOI: 10.1016/j.ophtha.2009.11.024

[40] Campochiaro PA, Brown DM, Pearson A et al. Sustained delivery fluocinolone acetonide vitreous inserts provide benefit for at least 3 years in patients with diabetic macular edema. *Ophthalmology* 2012;119(10):2125-2132. DOI: 10.1016/j.ophtha.2012.04.030

[41] Semenza GL. Vascular responses to hypoxia and ischemia. *Arterioscler Thromb Vasc Biol* 2010; 30: 648-652. DOI: 10.1161/ATVBAHA.108.181644

[42] Funatsu H, Yamashita H, Hori S. et al. Angiotensin II and vascular endothelial growth factor in the vitreous fluid of patients with diabetic macular edema and other retinal disorders. *Am J Ophthalmol* 2002;133:537-543.

[43] Aiello LP, Avery RL, Park JE. et al. Vascular endothelial growth factor in ocular fluid of patients with diabetic retinopathy and other retinal disorders. *N Engl J Med* 1994; 331:1480-1487.

[44] Miller JW, Le Couter J, Strauss EC, Ferrara N. Vascular endothelial growth factor a in intraocular vascular disease. *Ophthalmology* 2013; 120: 106-114 DOI: 10.1016/j.ophtha.2012.07.038

[45] Van der Reis MI, La Heij EC, Schouten JS et al. A systematic review of the adverse events of intravitreal anti-vascular endothelial growth factor injections. *Retina* 2011 Sep;31:1449-1469. DOI: 10.1097/IAE.0b013e3182278ab4.

[46] Nicholson BP, Schachat AP. A review of clinical trials of anti-VEGF agents for diabetic retinopathy. *Graefe's Arch Clin Exper Ophthalmol* 2010; 248(7): 915-930. DOI: 10.1007/s00417-010-1315-z.

[47] Nguyen QD, Shah SM, Khwaja AA et al. Two-year outcomes of the ranibizumab for edema of the macula in diabetes (READ-2) study. *Ophthalmology* 2010; 117: 2146-2151. DOI: 10.1016/j.ophtha.2010.08.016

[48] Schmidt Erfurth U, Lang GE, Holz FG et al. Three year outcomes of individualized ranibizumab treatment in patients with diabetic macular edema. The RESTORE extension study. Ahead of print. *Ophthalmology* 2014;121:1045-1053. DOI: 10.1016/j.ophtha.2013.11.041

[49] Elman MJ, Aiello LP, Beck RW et al. Randomized trial evaluating ranibizumab plus prompt or deferred laser or triamcinolone plus prompt laser for diabetic macular edema. *Ophthalmology* 2010;117:1064-1077.e35. DOI: 10.1016/j.ophtha.2014.08.047

[50] Elman MJ, Qin H, Aiello LP et al. Intravitreal ranibizumab for diabetic macular edema with prompt versus deferred laser treatment: three-year randomized trial results. *Ophthalmology* 2012; 119: 2312-2318. DOI: 10.1016/j.ophtha.2012.08.022

[51] Comparison of Age-related Macular Degeneration Treatments Trials (CATT) Research Group, Martin DF,Ferris FL et al. Ranibizumab and bevacizumab for treatment of neovascular age-related macular degeneration: two-year results. *Ophthalmology* 2012;119:1388-1398. DOI: 10.1016/j.ophtha.2012.03.053.

[52] Stefanini FR1, Arevalo JF, Maia M. Bevacizumab for the management of diabetic macular edema. *World J Diabetes* 2013;4:19-26. DOI:10.4239/wjd.v4.i2.19.

[53] Rajendram R, Fraser-Bell S, Kaines A, et al. A 2-year prospective randomized controlled trial of intravitreal bevacizumab or laser therapy (BOLT) in the management of diabetic macular edema: 24-month data: Report 3. *Arch Ophthalmol* 2012;130(8):972–979.

[54] DA VINCI Study Group. One-year outcomes of the DA VINCI study of VEGF trap-eye in eyes with diabetic macular edema. *Ophthalmology* 2012;119(8):1658–1665. DOI: 10.1016/j.ophtha.2012.02.010

[55] Heier J. Intravitreal aflibercept for diabetic macular edema: 12 month efficacy and safety results of phase 3, randomized, controlled VISTA-DME and VIVID-DME studies. 2014.

[56] Diana D. Visual and anatomic outcomes from the VISTA-DME and VIVID-DME studies of intravitreal aflibercept injection in diabetic macular edema patients with and without prior treatment for DME. 2014.

[57] Storey P, Dollin M, Garg SJ et al. Post-Injection Endophthalmitis Study Team. The role of topical antibiotic prophylaxis to prevent endophthalmitis after intravitreal injection. *Ophthalmology* 2014 Jan;121:283-289. DOI: 10.1016/j.ophtha.2013.08.037.

[58] ETDRS 1991: Early photocoagulation for diabetic retinopathy. ETDRS Report 9. Early Treatment Diabetic Retinopathy Study Research Group. *Ophthalmology* 1991;98(5): 766-785.

[59] Silva PS, Sun JK, Aiello LP et al. Role of steroids in the management of diabetic macular edema and proliferative diabetic retinopathy. *Sem Ophthalmol* 2009;24(2):93-99. DOI: 10.1080/08820530902800355.

[60] Mirshahi A, Roohipoor R, Lashay A et al. Bevacizumab-augmented retinal laser photocoagulation in proliferative diabetic retinopathy: a randomized double- masked clinical trial. *Eur J Ophthalmol* 2008;18(2):263-269.

[61] El Annan J, Carvounis PE. Current management of vitreous hemorrhage due to proliferative diabetic retinopathy. *Int Ophthalmol Clin* 2014;54:141-153. DOI: 10.1097/IIO. 0000000000000027.

[62] Martinez-Zapata MJ, Marti-Crvajal AJ, Evans JR et al. Anti-vascular endothelial growth factor for proliferative diabetic retinopathy. 2014;11. DOI: 10.1002/14651858.CD008721.pub2.

[63] Moradian S, Ahmadieh H, Malihi M. et al. Intravitreal Bevacizumab in active progressive proliferative diabetic retinopathy. *Graefe's Arch Clin Exper Ophthalmol.* 2008;246(12):1699-1705. DOI: 10.1007/s00417-008-0914-4.

[64] Ahmadieh H, Shoeibi N, Entezari M, Monshizadeh R. Intravitreal Bevacizumab for prevention of early postvitrectomy hemorrhage in diabetic patients: a randomized clinical trial. *Ophthalmology* 2010; 116:1943-1948. DOI: 10.1016/j.ophtha. 2009.07.001

[65] Shultz KL, Birnbaum AD, Goldsteir DA. Ocular disease in pregnancy. *Curr Opin Ophthalmol* 2005;16(5):308-314.

[66] Vestgaard M, Ringholm L, Laugesen CS et al. Pregnancy-induced sight- threatening diabetic retinopathy in women with type 1 diabetes. *Diabet Med* 2010; 27(4):431-435. DOI: 10.1111/j.1464-5491.2010.02958.x.

[67] Chew EY, Mills JL, Metzger BE et al. Metabolic control and progression of retinopathy. The Diabetic in Early Pregnancy Study. National Institute of Child Health and Human Development. Diabetes in Early Pregnancy Study. *Diabetes Care*1995;18(5): 631-637.

[68] Kastelan S, Tomic M, Pavan J,Oreskovic S. Maternal immune system adaptation to pregnancy – a potential influence on the course of diabetic retinopathy. *Reproduct Biol Endocrinol* 2010;8:124-128. DOI: 10.1186/1477-7827-8-124.

[69] Tarantola RM, Folk JC, Culver Boldt H, Mahajan VB. Intravitreal Bevacizumab during pregnancy. *Retina.* 2010; 30(9): 1405-1411. DOI: 10.1097/IAE.0b013e3181f57d58.

[70] Kim SJ, Equi R, Bressler NM. Analysis of macular edema after cataract surgery in patients with diabetes using optical coherence tomography. *Ophthalmology* 2007 May; 114:881-889.

[71] Ostri C, Lund-Andersen H, La Cour M et al. Phacoemulsification cataract surgery in a large cohort of diabetes patients: visual acuity outcomes and prognostic factors. *J Cataract Refract Surg* 2011;37:2006-2011. DOI: 10.1016/j.jcrs.2011.05.030.

[72] Diabetic Retinopathy Clinical Research Network Authors/Writing Committee, Baker CW, Almukhtar T, Stockdale C et al. Macular edema after cataract surgery in eyes without preoperative central-involved diabetic macular edema. *JAMA Ophthalmol* 2013;131:870-879. DOI: 10.1001/jamaophthalmol.2013.2313.

[73] O'Brien TP. Emerging guidelines for use of NSAID therapy to optimize cataract surgery patient care. *Curr Med Res Opin* 2005 Jul;21:1131-1137.

[74] Singh R, Alpern L, Sager D et al. Evaluation of nepafenac in prevention of macular edema followingcataract surgery in patients with diabetic retinopathy. *Clin Ophthalmol* 2012;6:1259-1269. DOI: 10.2147/OPTH.S31902.

[75] Cheema RA, Al- Mubarak MM, Amin YM et al. Role of combined cataract surgery and intravitreal Bevacizumab injection in preventing progression of diabetic retinopathy; prospective randomized study. *J Cataract Refract Surg* 2009;35:18-25. DOI: 10.1016/j.jcrs.2008.09.019

[76] Chen CH, Liu YC, Wu PC. The combination of intravitreal Bevacizumab and phacoemulsification surgery in patients with cataract and coexisting diabetic macular edema. *J Ocular Pharmacol Therapeut* 2009; 25,83-89. DOI: 10.1089/jop.2008.0068.

[77] Pollack A, Dotan S, Oliver M. Course of diabetic retinopathy following cataract surgery. *Brit J Ophthalmol* 1991;75(1):2-8.

[78] Hauser D, Katz H, Pokroy R. et al. Occurrence and progression of diabetic retinopathy after phacoemulsification cataract surgery. *J Cataract Refract Surg* 2004; 30(2): 428-432.

[79] Jaffe GJ, Burton TC, Kuhn E. et al. Progression of nonproliferative diabetic retinopathy and visual outcome after extracapsular cataract extraction and intraocular lens implantation. *Am J Ophthalmol* 1992; 114(4):448-456.

[80] Hayashi K, Igrarashi C, Hirata A et al. Changes in diabetic macular edema after phacoemulsification surgery. *Eye (London)*. 2009; 23(2): 386-389.

[81] Rashid S, Young LH. Progression of diabetic retinopathy and maculopathy afterphacoemulsification surgery. *Int Ophthalmol Clin/* 2010; 50(1): 155-166. *doi: 10.1097/IIO.0b013e3181c555cf.*

[82] Shah AS, Chen SH. Cataract surgery and diabetes. *Curr Opin Ophthalmol*. 2010:21(1): 4-9. doi: 10.1097/ICU.0b013e328333e9c1.

[83] Haddad NM, Sun JK, Silva PS et al. Cataract surgery and its complications in diabetic patients. *Rev Semin Ophthalmol* 2014;29:329-337. DOI: 10.3109/08820538.2014.959197.

[84] Chew EY, Benson WE, Remaley NA et al. Results after lens extraction in patients with diabetic retinopathy; early treatment diabetic retinopathy study report number 25. Arch Ophthalmol 1999:117(12):1600-1606.

Chapter 4

Complication of Type 1 Diabetes in Craniofacial and Dental Hard Tissue

Ippei Watari, Mona Aly Abbassy, Katarzyna Anna Podyma-Inoue and Takashi Ono

Additional information is available at the end of the chapter

http://dx.doi.org/10.5772/61885

Abstract

Diabetes mellitus (DM) is a chronic systemic disease arisen under the conditions when the body cannot produce enough insulin or cannot use it effectively. Type 1 diabetes is caused by an autoimmune reaction, where the body's defense system attacks the insulin-producing β-cells in the pancreas. Type 1 diabetes incidence has been rising all over the world, especially under the age of 15 years. There are strong premonitions of geographic difference; however, the overall annual increase in a number of affected population is estimated to be approximately 3%.

Under these circumstances, detailed understanding of the influence of type 1 diabetes on various organs is integrant. The systematic diseases have been seen to have a considerable effect on bone. As such, diabetes also exerts some degree of influence on bone in general. Hyperglycemia or impaired glucose metabolism has a number of detrimental effects on bone metabolism; for example, it is well documented that bone mass decreases and rate of bone fracture risk increases in type 1 diabetes patients. Nonetheless, there are few reports describing the influence of type 1 diabetes on hard tissue in craniofacial region.

From a dental clinical perspective, uncontrolled diabetic condition is thought to be one of the main causative factors of increased risk of inflammation and dental caries that lead to tooth loss and may also increase the risk of cardiovascular disease or preterm birth. However, there are only few reports focusing on type 1 diabetes complication in oral and maxillofacial region. Thus, in this chapter, we summarize the complication of type 1 diabetes in craniofacial hard tissue. Based on our previous data, type 1 diabetes lead to the retardant effects in cranium, mandible, and teeth during early growth period. This information is of critical importance not only for the better understanding of the type 1 diabetes complication in jaw or teeth but also for the development of efficient treatment and prevention of oral diseases in type 1 diabetes patients.

Keywords: Craniofacial complex, growth, type I diabetes, gestational diabetes

1. Introduction

Type 1 diabetes is a chronic and a complex autoimmune disease arisen primarily due to β-cell destruction. Historically, type 1 diabetes was considered as a disorder in children and adolescents, but now it is known that symptomatic onset of type 1 diabetes may occur at any age. Three major symptoms, polydipsia, polyphagia, and polyuria along with overt hyperglycemia, are a diagnostic hallmark in young type 1 diabetes patients. Exogenous insulin replacement is needed immediately after the onset of type 1 diabetes and should be kept throughout their lifetime for survival.

To prevent the diabetic complication, patients with type 1 diabetes require a strict control of blood glucose level.

Although type 1 diabetes can be diagnosed at any age, it is one of the most common chronic diseases of childhood. Its prevalence increases between the ages 5 and 7 years or near puberty [1].

It has been reported that the incidence of type 1 diabetes is increasing worldwide for several decades [2] and it is likely to have been most pronounced in children aged 4 years and younger [3]. If these trends continue, the total prevalence of people with type 1 diabetes will increase in the coming years [4].

A continuous hyperglycemia in type 1 diabetes leads to various chronic complications. Recently, official healthcare providers have paid more attention to the prevention of disabling chronic complications, such as diabetic retinopathy, nephropathy, neuropathy, and atherosclerosis with cardiovascular disease, and much more attention has been paid for adverse bone metabolism in type 1 diabetes. [5] In this review, we provide a brief overview on the effects of type 1 diabetes on both bone in general and hard tissue in craniofacial region.

2. General effects of type 1 diabetes on bone

The relation between diabetes and bone metabolism has been considered for a long time; however, many questions still remain hidden and unclear. Pathophysiology of diabetes arises from the insufficient insulin action, and such insulin action may have an influence on the bone metabolism directly or indirectly. Clinically, it is well known that type 1 and type 2 diabetes are involved in an increased risk of fractures [6, 7]; on the other hand, bone mineral density

(BMD) is decreased in type 1 diabetes than in type 2 diabetes [7]. The reasons for this discrepancy are not fully understood. Indeed both type 1 and type 2 diabetes are the same in terms of an abnormal glucose tolerance, but pathological condition is different. In this part, we discuss diabetic osteopenia in type 1 diabetes from the viewpoints of insulin deficiency and hyperglycemia.

2.1. Insulin deficiency and bone metabolism

It is widely recognized that bone volume and bone quality are decreased in type 1 diabetes patients, and it is thought that insulin has a pivotal role in bone formation [7]. In animal experiment, streptozotocin (STZ)-induced type 1 diabetes rat or mouse showed a decrease in bone volume (BV) and bone fragility by the decrease of bone formation [8–10].

In insulin receptor substrate-1 (IRS-1)-deficient mouse, osteoblast differentiation and function were impaired, and as a result, there is a decrease in BV [11].

Remarkable hyperglycemia exists with insulin deficiency in the type 1 diabetes model animals, and it seems to be thought that not only the insulin deficiency but also the hyperglycemic condition gives some influences on bone metabolism. On the other hand, it appears that decrease in anabolic action at the osteoblasts level in type 1 diabetes is the main cause of the bone metabolism disorder by serial animal experiments in which the disorder of glucose metabolism is slight under the normal breeding condition in IRS-1- or IRS-2-deficient mice. On the basis of these findings, one should consider the rise in onset, osteoporosis, and bone fracture frequency of the osteoporosis in type 1 diabetes mellitus depends on an osteoplasty disorder by the insulin deficiency.

2.2. Bone Mineral Density (BMD) in type 1 diabetes

In 1948, Albright and Reifenstein described for the first time the association between diabetes and reduced bone mass [12]. In 1976, Levin et al. demonstrated that almost 50% of the patients with type 1 diabetes had a reduction of BMD at the wrist [13]. Since then, many papers have been published. BMD seems to be reduced in patients with type 1 diabetes in most [14–17], but not all [18, 19]. The studies concerning the bone metabolism in type 1 diabetes can be categorized into two groups: 1) studies evaluating bone metabolism in diabetic children and adolescents who did not reach the peak of bone mass yet and 2) studies evaluating bone metabolism in adults who developed type 1 diabetes after having reached peak of bone mass.

It seems to be difficult to study bone metabolism in such population as children/adolescents whose skeleton is still in the way of growing. Moreover, the majority of studies included the children/adolescents at different stage of puberty and, therefore, at different stages of acquisition of bone mass. This probably has been one of the main reasons for the lack of concordant results about the impact of diabetes on growing bones.

Some reports showed no differences in BMD between type 1 diabetic children/adolescents and their peer without diabetes [20–26]. However, in other studies, low bone mineral content (BMC) and low BMD both at spine and at femoral neck in type 1 diabetic children/adolescents

[27–33] have been described. Moreover, some longitudinal studies demonstrated a significant reduction of either lumber spine or femoral neck BMD in diabetic patients after 2–4 years of follow-up, despite normal BMD at baseline [20, 23]. Therefore, it seems that type 1 diabetes, appeared in childhood, may alter the acquisition of bone mass that can be registered in youth ages or later in adult life.

Indeed, the majority of studies, performed on the type 1 diabetes adults, consistently showed a reduction of BMD either at lumbar spine and/or at femur [34, 35, 36–40]. Only a few studies [41–43], which were conducted on small groups of diabetic patients (less than 40 cases), were discordant. Vestergaard et al. [44] having analyzed 80 studies regarding bone density in diabetes has proved in his meta-analysis that type 1 diabetes patients have lower BMD than the people without diabetes. Frequency of reduced BMD in type 1 diabetes varies largely from 3 to 40% [36–40]. Eller-Vainicher et al. [45] reported that about 30% of 175 type 1 diabetes patients had low bone mass (osteopenia/osteoporosis) at spine and/or femur, which was significantly higher in comparison with healthy controls.

2.3. Fracture risk in type 1 diabetes

In type 1 diabetes patients, the frequency of lifetime fractures at any site has been reported to be increased as compared to counterparts without diabetes. The meta-analysis of Vestergaard et al. [44] demonstrated a 6.94-fold increased risk of hip fracture in type 1 diabetes. Further, *Zhukouskaya et al.* [45] reported that type 1 diabetes patients were found to have an increased prevalence of asymptomatic vertebral fractures as well, which have been observed in 25% of diabetic subjects. In conclusion, there is strong evidence that bones in type 1 diabetes patients are characterized by poor mineralization and smaller and thinner size with reduced bone strength and quality, which can lead to a higher fracture incidence at any site, predominantly at femoral neck.

2.4. Association between hyperglycemia and bone metabolism in diabetes

Type 1 diabetes is caused by absolute lack of insulin, and insulin has anabolic effect on bone. However, not only insulin but also hyperglycemia has some influence on the bone metabolism. In in vivo study, it is difficult to evaluate the influence on bone metabolism by hyperglycemia or insulin deficiency separately, so the influence of hyperglycemia on bone is considered at a cell level mainly.

In an experiment of osteoblastic cell, it was reported that the differentiation and function of osteoblastic cell were suppressed under osmolality-adjusted hyperglycemic condition [46].

In our previous experiment using MC3T3-E1 cell line, osteoblastic cells were cultured in medium containing normal (5.6 mM) or high (10, 20, or 30 mM) glucose with or without bone morphogenic protein 2 (BMP-2). Runx2 mRNA expression, which is a key transcription factor associated with osteoblast differentiation, was affected by glucose concentration and culture duration independently of the absence or presence of BMP-2 in the culture. (Fig. 1) [47]. Moreover, we could find both GLP-1 receptor (GLP-1R) and GIP receptor (GIPR) m RNA expression in osteoblastic cell first time ever (Fig. 2), and mRNA expression level of GLP-1R and GIPR were regulated by glucose concentrations in cells undergoing the differentiation induced by BMP-2 (Figs. 3, 4). GLP-1 or GIP belong to the incretin family. They both play important roles in regulating insulin secretion from pancreatic β-cells. GIPR and GLP-1R, the receptors of GIP and GLP-1, are expressed in various tissues, with a significant amount expressed in pancreas. Previous reports showed that GIPR is expressed in osteoblastic cells, but no study regarding GLP-1R expression had been conducted [48]. Although osteoblastic cells were thought to express a functional receptor for GLP-1, there is no direct evidence for the mRNA and protein expression of GLP-1R in these cells. GIP is known to have direct effects on bone, whereas the effects of GLP-1 on bone metabolism are mediated by thyroid hormone. [49] Our RT-PCR analysis revealed that MC3T3-E1 cells express GLP-1R and GIPR, suggesting that GLP-1 may directly affect bone, similar to GIP (Fig. 4). GLP-1R and GIPR are well-known G protein-coupled receptor (GPCR) and are potential targets for drug discovery [47]. It has been reported that the administration of insulin and thiazolidinediones increases fracture risk, whereas inhibitors of dipeptidyl peptidase-4 (DPP-4) were associated with reduced fracture risk. DPP-4 inactivates GLP-1, and its inhibitors improve glycemic control in patients with type 2 diabetes by preventing incretin degradation [50]. These findings show that GLP-1R links bone metabolism and glucose metabolism in osteoblasts and that GLP-1 might be a potential therapeutic target in bone diseases.

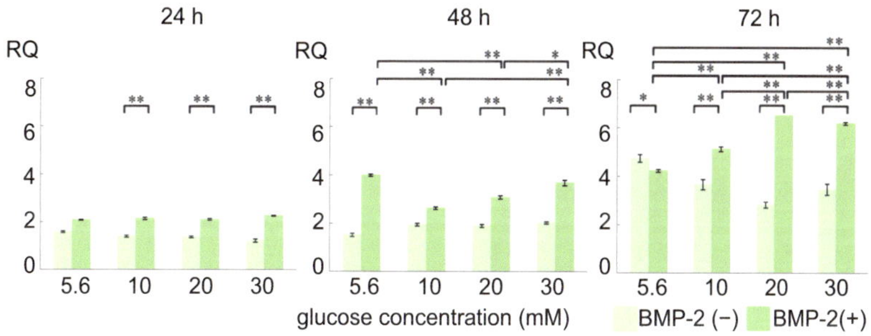

Figure 1. Effects of the glucose concentration on Runx2 mRNA expression. MC3T3-E1 cells were cultured in medium containing 5.6 (normal), or 10, 20, and 30 mM (high) concentrations of glucose in the absence or presence of bone morphogenetic protein-2 (BMP-2). Runx2 mRNA expression was determined after 24, 48, and 72 h of culture. Values are the means ± standard error of the mean (SEM) (n = 4/group). *$P < 0.05$ and **$P < 0.01$.

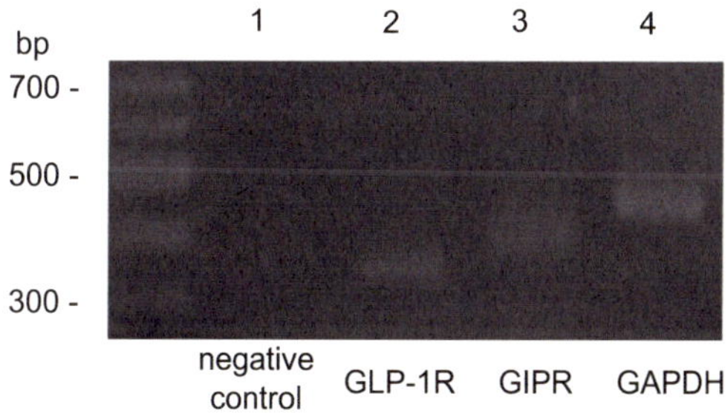

Figure 2. Reverse transcriptase-polymerase chain reaction (RT-PCR) analysis of glucagon-like peptide-1 receptor (GLP-1R) and glucose-dependent insulinotropic polypeptide receptor (GIPR) mRNA expression in MC3T3-E1 cells. Lane 1, negative control; lane 2, GLP-1R (337 bp); lane 3, GIPR (382 bp); lane 4, GAPDH (452 bp).

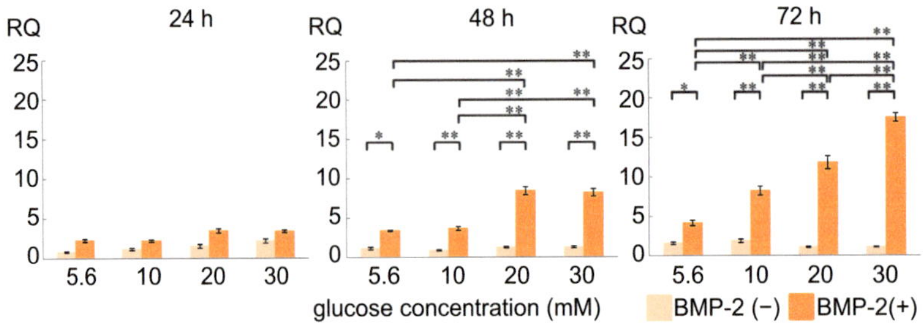

Figure 3. Effects of the glucose concentration on glucagon-like peptide-1 receptor (GLP-1R) mRNA expression. MC3T3-E1 cells were cultured in medium containing 5.6 (normal), or 10, 20 and 30 mM (high) concentrations of glucose in the absence or presence of bone morphogenetic protein-2 (BMP-2). GLP-1R mRNA expression after 24, 48, and 72 h of culture. Values are the means ± standard error of the mean (SEM) ($n = 4$/group). $^{*}P < 0.01$.

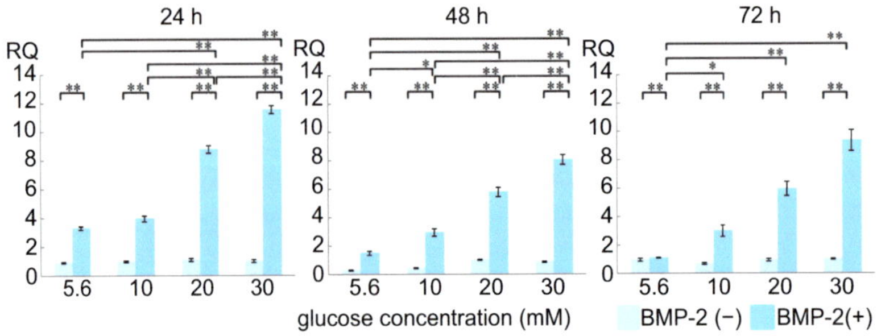

Figure 4. Effects of glucose concentration on glucose- dependent insulinotropic polypeptide receptor (GIPR) mRNA expression. MC3T3-E1 cells were cultured in medium containing 5.6 (normal), or 10, 20, and 30 mM (high) concentrations of glucose in the absence or presence of bone morphogenetic protein-2 (BMP-2). GIPR mRNA expression after 24, 48, and 72 h of culture. Values are the means ± standard error of the mean (SEM) ($n = 4$/group). $^{*}P < 0.01$.

3. Effect of type 1 diabetes on craniofacial complex

Diabetes is one of the systemic diseases affecting a considerable number of patients worldwide [51]. Numerous clinical and experimental studies on the complications of diabetes have demonstrated extensive alterations in bone and mineral metabolism, linear growth, and body composition [52]. As we mentioned in the previous section, depletion of insulin in type 1 diabetes causes a reduction of bone composition, delay in fracture healing, and reduction of BMD in general. A long list of literature was dedicated to study the influence or complications of type 1 diabetes on general bones. However, there are few reports discussing the effects of type 1 diabetes on the craniofacial complex which is regulated by hormones, nutrients, mechanical forces, and various peripheral growth factors.

In craniofacial region, it is well known that bone metabolism in growth period is really intricate because there are mosaic growth sites where bones grow at different rates or mature at different times, which also depend on each individual's growth stage, and the response to growth disruption is much more complicated than that of the appendicular skeleton. There are a few studies diabetes may significantly affect the bone remodeling process which is observed during treatments involving the application of mechanical or functional force to the craniofacial complex and the teeth as those applied during orthodontic tooth movement. Moreover, it is likely that the type 1 diabetes may have altered the growth of patients due to insulin deficiency and consequently led to skeletal mutation is it mutation or maturation?

Type 1 diabetes is well recognized in the endocrine disorders,, and a peak of onset is concentrated in childhood and adolescence, characterized by hyperglycemia as a cardinal biochemical feature that leads to several impairment of physical and emotional developments. There are some reports focusing on the altered bone remodeling in type 1 diabetes, which indicates the reduction of osteoblast activity or function. Bone mass decrease and rate of bone fracture risk increase have been often seen in type 1 diabetes patients. Impaired glucose metabolism results in adverse effects on bone metabolism, especially in type 1 diabetes patients who suffer from decreased bone mineral density (BMD) and increased risk of fractures. The pathophysiological mechanisms of increased risk of fracture in diabetes patients are divided into two reasons: osteopenia caused by decreased BMD and increased risk of fall and traumas caused by peripheral diabetic neuropathy. However, there are few reports about hard tissue in craniofacial region, in other words, cranium, maxilla, mandible, and teeth.

The aim of this chapter is to discuss the complexity of the dento-alveolar system and how it was affected by type 1 diabetes.

3.1. Effect of type 1 diabetes on bone in craniofacial region

There are two processes of bone formation: "intramembranous ossification" and "endochondral ossification." Endochondral ossification is a cartilage bone formation and it occurs in a replacement process within the cartilage models of the embryo and infant. Intramembranous bone forms through the activation of the osteoblastic cell or specialized bone forming cell in one of the layers of the fetal-connective tissue. The bones of the cranial vault, the face, and the clavicle are formed by the style of intramembranous ossification. All the other bones are formed in the manner of cartilage ossification. The bones formed by intramembranous ossification are the mandible, the maxilla, the premaxilla, the frontal bone, the palatine bone, the squamous part of temporal bone, the zygomatic bone, the medial plate of the pterygoid process, the vomer, the tympanic part of the temporal bone, the nasal bone, the lacrimal bone, and the parietal bone. The original pattern of intramembranous bone changes with progressive maturative growth when these bones begin to adapt to environmental influences. This accounts for deformities due to malfunction, disease, and other environmental factor [53].

3.2. Causes of general growth problems

It is thought that growth disturbance can be associated with specific anatomic or functional defects. Some kinds of endocrinal or metabolic disorders are known to cause a systemic growth disorder. Also, genetic, nutritional, or environmental factor can be the causes of growth disturbance. Disturbances in somatic growth show themselves in retardation or acceleration of the skeletal system, including the facial and cranial bones. Causes of growth problems usually fall into the following categories [54]:

- familial short stature;
- constitutional growth delay with delayed adolescence or delayed maturation;
- illness that affects the whole body (systemic disease);
- endocrine disease (hormonal disorder); and
- congenital problems in the tissues where growth occurs.

3.3. Effect of type 1 diabetes on bone and growth

Concerning juvenile diabetes, previous report about hand-wrist radiographs [55]. showed that usually, there is a delay in the development of appearance or ossification center of the carpal bone. These defects seem to occur twice as frequently in boys than in girls, and the total incidence of juvenile diabetes patients with abnormalities and developmental disorders was 24.3%.There was also a delay in the growth of bone, in 51% of diabetic males and in 60% of diabetic females. The trend of growth retardation in bone was large. The longer the disease duration of diabetes, the shorter the bone growth will be. Bone mass reduction in diabetic patients has been explained by the decrease in the proliferative capacity of fibroblasts. In addition, premature aging of all cells has been suggested as the basis for diabetes problems, which is believed to lead to early osteopenia. The yearly bone loss was reported to be 1.35% in patients with type 1 diabetes [56]. Moreover, reduction rate of bone mineral, along with the condition worsened in diabetes, was significantly faster despite of an increase in insulin dosage, when compared with patients with unchanged or improved insulin secretion. It was considered that exogenous insulin administration cannot fully compensate for the decrease in the endogenous insulin secretion. In addition, according to these studies, the bone resorption in patients with type 1 diabetes were increased, and vitamin D_3 deficiency associated with the disease were not observed. Vertebral bone density has been studied in type 1 diabetic children [56]. In diabetic children, it has been found that the cortical bone density decreases slightly but significantly compared with control. The decrease in the cortical bone mineral density in diabetes did not correlate with age, gender, the duration of the diabetes, or glycosylated hemoglobin concentration. These results suggested that in children with uncomplicated type 1 diabetes, decreased vertebral bone density is a minor abnormality that affects only cortical bone [55].

3.4. Outline of studying the effect of type 1 diabetes on craniofacial growth

To examine the dynamic bone metabolism and structure of craniofacial bone in diabetes, it is critically important in understanding the growth aspect and bone metabolism of the mandible. The next parts of this chapter are trying to focus on the following points:

1. The effects of juvenile diabetes on general craniofacial growth and skeletal maturation.
2. Analysis of the pattern of association between craniofacial morphology and skeletal maturation.
3. Determination of the mineral apposition rate and the bone formation rate in diabetic rat mandible using histomorphometric analysis.
4. Analysis of the diabetic effects on tooth (enamel and dentin formation).

3.5. Experimental rat model for type 1 diabetes

It is well known that the streptozotocin-induced diabetic rat and the spontaneously diabetic BioBreeding rat were used as experimental type 1 diabetic models [57]. Pathogenesis of altered bone formation in long bones after inducing type 1 diabetes with streptozotocin (STZ) has been well documented [58, 59]. Streptozotocin-induced diabetes mellitus (STZ-DM) caused by the destruction of pancreatic β-cells and is similar to type 1 diabetes in human. It is characterized by mild-to-moderate hyperglycemia, glucosuria, polyphagia, hypoinsulinemia, hyperlipidemia, and weight loss. STZ-DM also exhibits many of the complications observed in human DM including enhanced susceptibility to infection and cardiovascular disease, retinopathy, alterations in angiogenesis, delayed wound healing, diminished growth factor expression, and reduced bone formation. [60].

3.6. Induction of type 1 diabetic condition in animal experiment

We studied various changes on craniofacial hard tissue under DM condition using streptozotocin (STZ)-induced DM rat model. Three-week-old male Wistar rats (n = 12) were used for this study. They were randomly divided into two groups, the control group and the diabetes group (DM group), and each group consists of six rats. The rats in the control group were injected intraperitoneally with a single dose of 0.1M sodium citrate buffer (pH 4.5), while the rats in the DM group were injected intraperitoneally with a single dose of citrate buffer containing 60 mg/kg body weight of STZ (Sigma Chemical Co., St. Louis, MO, USA) [58, 61–63]. All animals were fed on standard rodent diet (Rodent Diet CE-2; Japan Clea Inc., Shizuoka, Japan) with free access to water. Body weights, the presence of glucose in urine, and blood glucose levels were recorded on days 0, 2, 7, 14, 21, and 28 after STZ injection. Diabetes condition was determined by the presence of glucose in urine and blood. The urine of the rats was tested using reagent strips (Uriace Ga; TERUMO) [64, 65]. Blood samples of the rats were obtained via vein puncture of a tail vein, and blood glucose levels were determined using a glucometer (Ascensia Brio; Bayer Medical). Rats with a positive urine test and a blood glucose level greater than 200 mg/dl were considered as diabetic. Time course of the animal experiment is shown in Fig. 5.

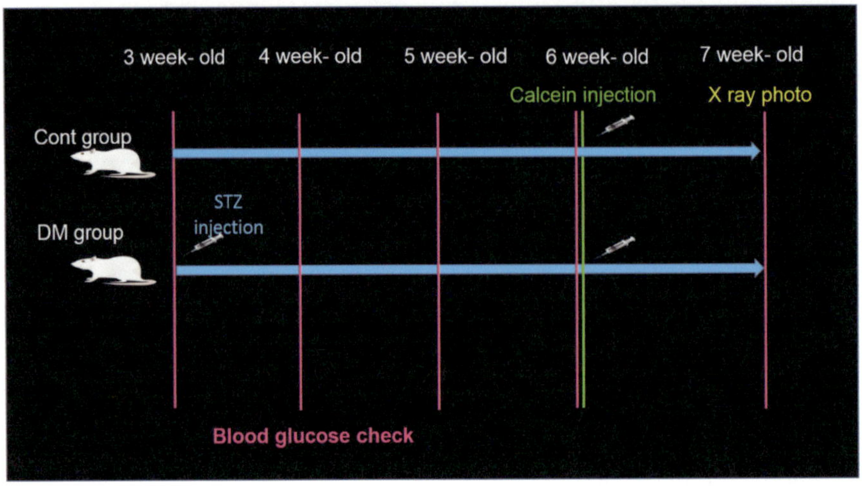

Figure 5. The time schedule of experiment

3.7. Evaluating the effect of type 1 diabetes on craniofacial growth in rat

Cephalometric analysis

Cephalometric measurements are still one of the most widely spread diagnostic aids crucial for the diagnosis of various abnormalities in the craniofacial complex [66].

The protocol for examining the cephalometric measurements in Type 1 diabetic rats involved the following steps:

1. Prior to each radiographic session, the rats were anesthetized with diethyl ether and intraperitoneally injected with 8% chloral hydrate using 0.5 ml/100 g of body weight.

2. After anesthesia, the rats were placed in the same way using specially designed apparatus to maintain standardized head posture and contact with the film (SGP-3; Mitsutoyo, Tokyo, Japan) where the head of each rat was fixed firmly with a pair of ear rods oriented vertically to the sagittal plane, and the incisors were fixed into a plastic ring. The settings of lateral and dorsoventral cephalometric radiographs were 50/55 kVp, 15/10 mA, and 20/60-sec impulses, respectively [68].

3. Then, a 10-mm steel calibration rod was incorporated into the clear acrylic table on which the animals were positioned for the radiographs.

All the radiographs were developed and scanned at high resolution by the same operator (Fig. 6). The cephalometric landmarks were derived from previous studies on rodents [68–70]. The selected linear measurements were then obtained (Table 1). To ensure reliability and reproducibility of each measurement, each distance was digitized twice and the two values were averaged. In our studies, evaluation of the craniofacial growth of diabetic rats at the age of 7 weeks was carried out using lateral and dorsoventral cephalometric radiographs. All of the data in each experiment were confirmed for the normal distribution; that is, Student's t-test

http://dx.doi.org/10.5772/61885

was used to compare the mean of each data recorded in the control group and in the DM group. All statistical analyses were performed at a 5% significance level using statistic software (v. 10; SPSS, Chicago, IL, USA).

Neurocranium	**Mandible**
Po–N: total skull length	Go–Mn: posterior corpus length
Po–E: cranial vault length	Ml–Il: anterior corpus length
Ba–E: total cranial base length	Co–Il: total mandibular length
So–E: anterior cranial base length	Co–Gn: ramus height
Ba–CB1: occipital bone length	**Transverse X-ray**
CB1′–CB2: sphenoid bone length	Go1–Go2: bigonial width
Ba–So: posterior cranial base length	C1–C2: maximum cranial width
Po–Ba: posterior neurocranium height	P1–P2: palatal width
Viscerocranium	Z1–Z2: bizygomatic width
E–N: nasal length	
Mu2–Iu: palate length	
CB2–Iu: midface length	
E–Mu1: viscerocranial height	

Table 1. Measurements of craniofacial skeleton

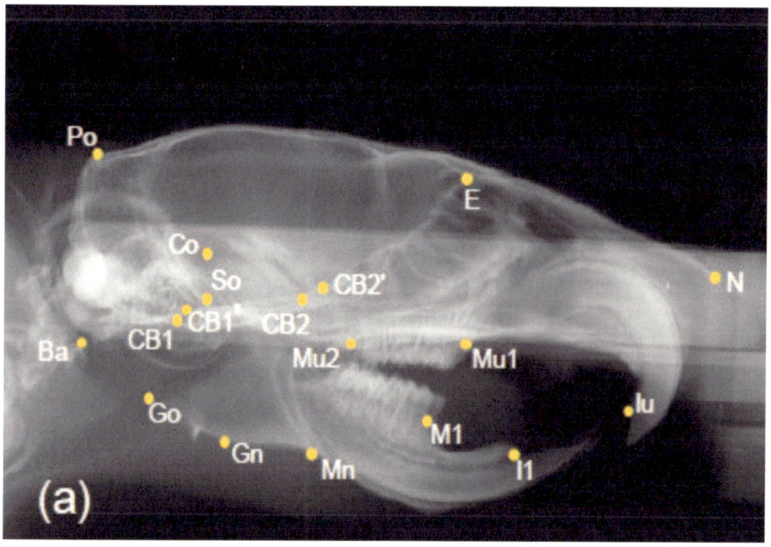

Figure 6. Location of lateral cephalometric points on radiographs: (a) sagittal

3.7.1. *Changes in the total skull*

The size of total skull, denoted by Po-N, was found to be significantly smaller in the DM group than in the control group (Fig. 7).

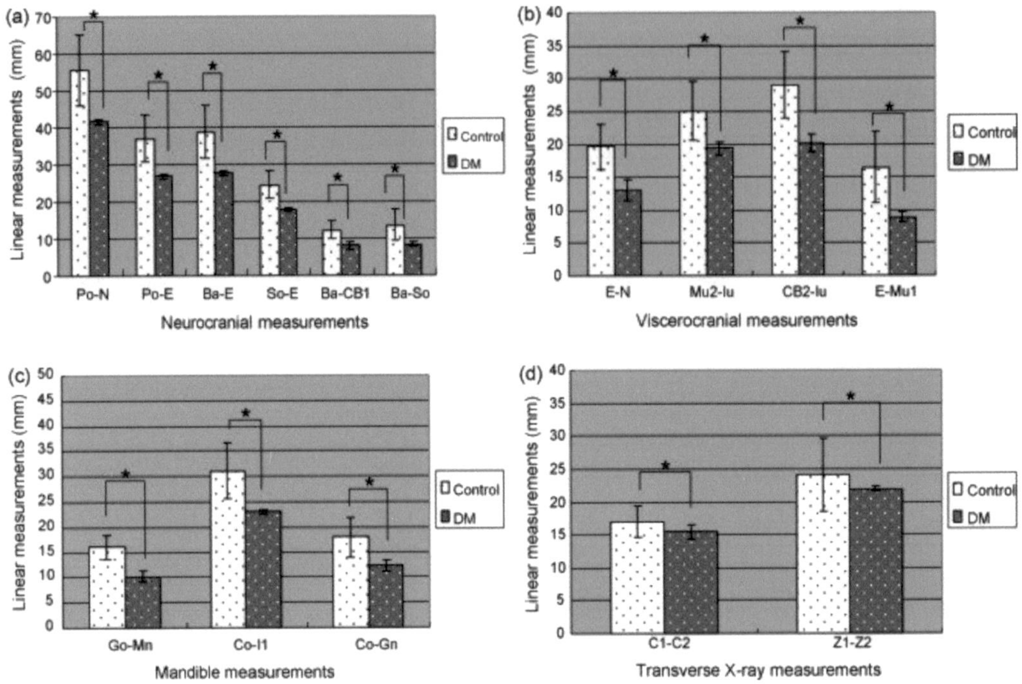

Figure 7. (A) Changes in the neurocranial measurements of the control and type 1 diabetes (DM) group. All the significant measurements are shown in this figure. Values are mean ± S.D. Significant differences between the two groups are marked with asterisks ($P < 0.05$). (B) Changes in the viscerocranial measurements of the control and DM groups. All the viscerocranial measurements are significant. Values are mean ± S.D. Significant differences between the two groups are marked with asterisks ($P < 0.05$). (C) Changes in the mandible measurements of the control and DM groups. Values are mean ± S.D. Significant differences between the two groups are marked with asterisks ($P < 0.05$). (D) Changes in the transverse X-ray measurements of the control and DM groups. Two measurements in the transverse X-ray were significant. Values are mean ± S.D. Significant differences between the two groups are marked with asterisks ($P < 0.05$).

3.7.2. *Changes observed in the Neurocranium*

Cranial vault length (Po-E), total cranial base length (Ba-E), anterior cranial base length (SoE), occipital bone length (Ba-CB1), and posterior cranial base length (Ba-So) were significantly shorter in DM group (Fig. 7), while the other dimensions showed no significant differences.

3.7.3. *Changes in the Viscerocranium*

All measurements of the viscerocranium, including the nasal length (E-N), palatal length (Mu2-Iu), midface length (CB2-Iu), and viscerocranial height (E-Mu1), showed a statistically significant decrease in DM group (Fig. 7).

3.7.4. Changes in the Mandible

In the DM group, the posterior corpus length (Go-Mn), total mandibular length (Co-Il), and the ramus height (Co-Gn) were significantly shorter than in the control group (Fig. 7); on the other hand, there were no statistical differences in the remaining dimensions.

3.8. Histomorphometric analysis of mandible

3.8.1. Fluorescent dyes used for double labeling in histomorphometric analysis

Fluorochromes are calcium-binding substances that are preferentially taken up at the site of active mineralization of bone known as the calcification front, thus labeling sites of new bone formation. They are detected using fluorescent microscopy on undecalcified sections. Labeling bones with fluorochrome markers provides a means to study the dynamics of bone formation. The rate and extent of bone deposition and resorption can be determined using double- and triple-fluorochrome labeling sequences. The sequential use of fluorochromes of clearly contrasting colors permits a more detailed record of events relating to calcification. Fluorochromes commonly used in mammals include tetracycline, calcein green, xylenol orange, alizarin red, and hematoporphyrin. Calcein gives bright green fluorescence when combined with calcium [71].

3.8.2. Calcein administrations and sections preparation

The detection of the double labeling involves the following steps:

- Rats are subcutaneously injected with 50 mg/kg body weight calcein fluorescent marker on day 21 and day 28 after STZ injection [72]. The time difference between the two injections was one week to be able to compare the amount of bone formed during this period (Fig. 8).
- All animals were sacrificed by transcardiac perfusion under deep anesthesia using 4% paraformaldehyde in 0.1 M phosphate buffer (pH 7.4).
- Mandibles were dissected and fixed in the same solution for 24 h and embedded in polystyrene resin (Rigolac; Nisshin EM Co. Ltd., Tokyo, Japan).
- Undermineralized ground frontal sections were processed to show the crown and both apices of buccal and lingual roots of the lower second molar [72].

3.8.3. Method of analysis of "Mineral Appositional Rate" and "Bone Formation Rate"

The bone around the lower second molar is centrally located within the mandibular arch, and the parallel alignment of the buccal and lingual roots is used as a precise reference when frontal sections are produced [73]. To conduct the histomorphometric analysis, it is essential to use a digitizing morphometry system to measure bone formation indices. The system consists of a confocal laser scanning microscope (LSM510; Carl Zeiss Co. Ltd., Jena, Germany) and a morphometry program (LSM Image Browser; Carl Zeiss Co. Ltd., Jena, Germany). Bone formation indices of the periosteal surfaces of the alveolar/jaw bone include mineral apposition

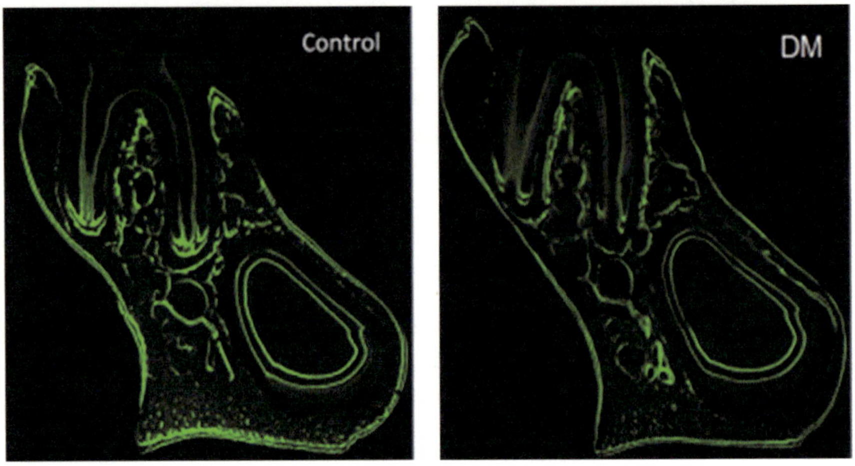

Figure 8. Frontal sections of the rat's mandibular second molar area. Control, control rat; DM, type 1 diabetes rat. Fluorescent labeling on the periosteal surface indicates new bone formation.

rate (μm/day) and bone formation rate (μm^3/μm^2/day), according to the standard nomenclature described by Parfitt and colleagues [74]. The calcein-labeled surface (CLS, in mm) is calculated as the sum of the length of double labels plus one half of the length of single labels (sL) along the entire endosteal or periosteal bone surfaces; that is, CLS = dL + 0.5sL [75]. The mineral apposition rate (MAR, in μm/day) is determined by dividing the mean of the width of the double labels by the interlabel time (7 days). The bone formation rate (BFR) is calculated by multiplying MAR by CLS [76]. Based on the reference line along the long axis of the buccal root, the area superior to the root apex was considered as an alveolar bone, while the area inferior to the root apex was considered as the jaw bone. The lingual side of the bone was excluded, because the existence of the incisor root might influence bone formation. The periosteal surfaces of the mandible were divided into four regions for analysis (Fig. 9).

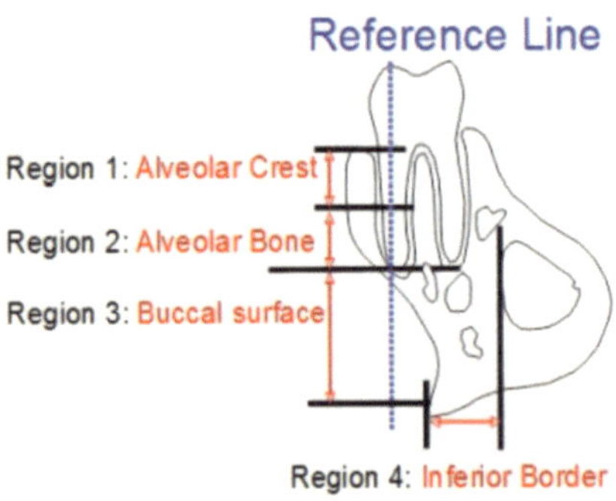

Figure 9. Schematic drawing of observation regions for dynamic bone histomorphometry. The periosteal surfaces were delimited into four areas: alveolar crest (region 1), alveolar bone (region 2), buccal surface of the jaw bone (region 3), and inferior border of the jaw bone (region 4).

3.8.4. Hitromorphometric indices

The obtained results in our study showed that in the alveolar bone (region 2), there was a significant decrease in the MAR (Fig. 10A) and the BFR (Fig. 10B) recorded in the DM group compared to the control group. However, in the alveolar crest (region 1), the MAR and the BFR in the control and the DM groups were not significantly different ($P < 0.05$). In the buccal surface (region 3) and inferior borders (region 4) of the jaw bone, the MAR (Fig. 10A) and BFR (Fig. 10B) were significantly suppressed compared with those in the control group ($P < 0.05$). Most of the periosteal surfaces in the mandibular regions of the control group showed significantly higher values recorded for the mineral apposition rate and the bone formation rate when compared to the DM group. These results agree with the previous studies that recorded diminished lamellar bone formation in DM rats' femur and may suggest an association between the DM condition and the decreased number and function of osteoblasts [61]. The alveolar crest region was the only region that did not show a significant difference in the MAR and the BFR parameters between the two groups; this may be attributed to the unique nature of this region exhibiting a highly intensive bone remodeling process especially during the teeth eruption that decreases toward the base of the socket [77]; however, further studies are needed to elaborate the detailed pattern of bone growth at the alveolar crest region.

3.9. Evaluating the type 1 diabetic effects on tooth

Type 1 diabetes exhibits various detrimental alterations on bones, and mineral metabolism [52, 58, 75]. However, there is scant information available on the possible effects exerted by the diabetic condition on tooth development and mineral content. Various clinical studies reported high caries prevalence in diabetic children when compared with healthy controls [78]. Previous studies suggested that the aforementioned increase in caries prevalence associated with type 1 diabetes may be due to alteration in the salivary gland functions resulting in decreased salivary flow. Alternative speculations were that type 1 diabetes produced increased salivary glucose levels which may have increased permeability of the parotid gland basement membrane to the elevated blood glucose. Understanding the factors contributing to the increased caries susceptibility of young patients suffering from the diabetic condition, especially young orthodontic patients who have high probability for the development of caries during their orthodontic treatment, may help dentists to plan suitable strategies for protecting such patients against the expected caries challenges. Moreover, it is of prime importance for dentists and orthodontists to explore any factors that might affect the dental tissues growth and thus the size of the teeth, which has a strong impact on the orthodontic treatment planning. Our study has employed the non-destructive micro-computed tomography (micro-CT) to examine the influence of induced type 1 diabetes on enamel and dentine mineral density and thickness using an experimental rat model. Micro-CT uses a focused beam to provide higher resolution on small samples in vitro. This method has been frequently used in experiments exploring bone and is considered as a promising technique for the assessment of tooth mineral density. In addition, a histomorphometric study was conducted to determine the effect of the type 1 diabetes condition on dentine formation and dentine mineral apposition rates in the continuously growing lower incisors of Wistar rats. This is an appropriate model for examining the

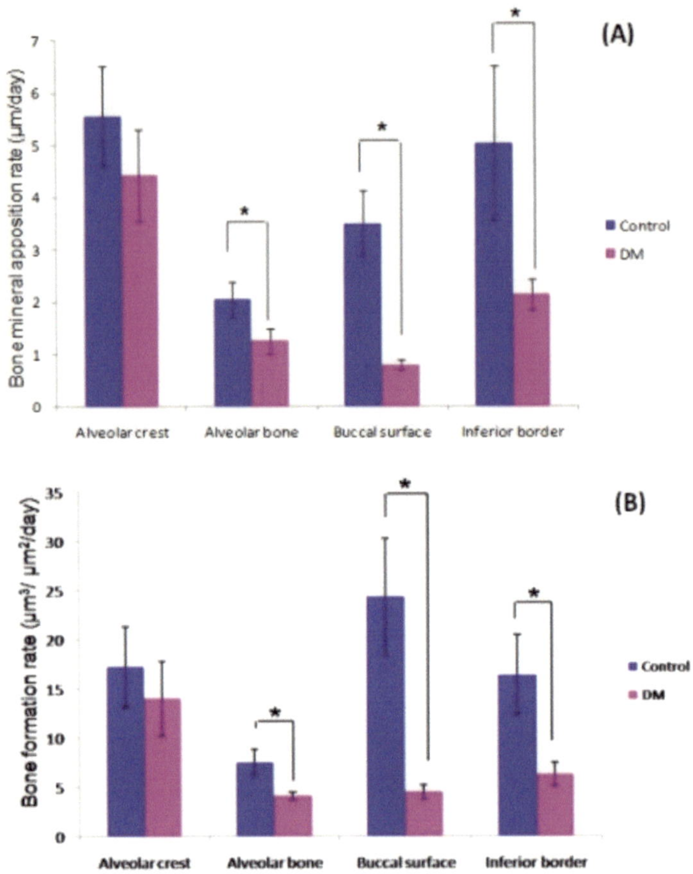

Figure 10. (A) Changes in the mineral apposition rate (MAR) of the mandible between the control group (red columns) and the type 1 diabetes mellitus (DM) group (blue columns). Alveolar crest (region 1, upper half of the tooth root, near the tooth crown). Alveolar bone (region 2, lower half of the tooth root, near the root apex). Buccal surface of the jaw bone (region 3). Inferior border of the jaw bone (region 4). The data are expressed as means ± S.D.; $n = 5$ for each group. Significantly different from controls, with $^*P < 0.05$. (B) Changes in the bone formation rate (BFR/BS) of the mandible between the control group and the DM group. Alveolar crest (region 1, upper half of the tooth root, near the tooth crown). Alveolar bone (region 2, lower half of the tooth root, near the root apex). Buccal surface of the jaw bone (region 3). Inferior border of the jaw bone (region 4). The data are expressed as means ± S.D.; $n = 5$ for each group. Significantly different from controls, with $^*P < 0.05$. In the buccal surface (region 3) and inferior borders (region 4) of the jaw bone, the MAR (Fig. 4A) and the BFR (Fig. 4B) are significantly suppressed compared with those in the control group ($P < 0.05$).

effects of different factors on the development of hard tissues. The tested null hypotheses in this study were that the type 1 diabetes condition will not adversely affect thickness, mineral density, and the rate of tissue formation and mineral apposition in enamel and dentine.

3.9.1. Calcein administration and section preparation for tooth observation

Rats were subcutaneously injected with calcein fluorescent marker (50 mg/kg body weight) on day 21 and day 28 after STZ injection. All animals were anesthetized and sacrificed by transcardiac perfusion by 4% paraformaldehyde in 0.1 M phosphate buffer (pH 7.4). The right mandibles were removed and fixed in the same solution. After being embedded in polystyrene resin (Rigolac; Nisshin EM Co. Ltd., Tokyo, Japan), undemineralized ground mesial sections were cut using water-cooled diamond saw microtome (1600 Microtome; Leitz Wetzlar, Germany) parallel to the long axis of the rat molars just 2 mm to the mesial surface of the first lower molar crown; the distal second cut was done 2 mm distal to the crown of the first molar. The specimen mesial surface was then ground flat with water-cooled silicon carbide discs (600- and 1200-grade papers; Buehler) until it was possible to observe the two mesial canals and two mesial pulp chamber horns of the first molar. The ground mesial surface was glued on a glass slide, and the same grinding procedures were repeated from the distal surface until we can observe the two mesial canals and two mesial pulp horns of the first molar from the distal side. The obtained specimen is then wet-polished using diamond paste (1 mm; Buehler) to obtain a highly polished surface.

3.9.2. Analysis of histomorphometric indices of tooth

Dentine formation indices in control and type 1 diabetes groups were determined in the crown analogue area parallel to the long axis of the mesial surface of the first molar. A digitizing morphometry system was used to measure the dentine formation indices. The system consisted of a confocal laser scanning microscope (LSM510; Carl Zeiss Co. Ltd., Jena, Germany) and a morphometry program (LSM Image Browser; Carl Zeiss Co. Ltd., Germany). Dentine formation indices included dentine mineral apposition rate (mm/day) and dentine formation rate ($\mu m^3/\mu m^2$/day). The method for the calculation of bone indices was modified from a method described by Parfitt et al. [74] The calcein-labeled dentine surface (CLS, in mm) was calculated as the sum of the length of double labels (dL) plus one half of the length of single labels (sL) along the entire dentine surface; that is, CLS = dL + 0.5sL [17]. The mineral apposition rate (MAR, in μm/day and in μm^2/day) was determined by dividing the mean of the width of the double labels by the interlabel time (7 days). The dentine formation rate (DFR) was calculated by multiplying MAR by CLS [18]. For the measurements of mineral apposition rate, the average of 3 inter-label widths at a 100-μm interval was calculated for each sample.

Green fluorescent lines labeled with calcein fluorescent marker at two different time points showed that dentine formation took place between day 21 and day 28 in the control and type 1 diabetes groups (Fig. 11A and B). In the type 1 diabetes group, there were significant decreases in both mineral apposition and dentine formation rates (Fig. 11C and D) when compared to control group ($P < 0.05$).

Furthermore, our micro-CT results (details of method not shown) revealed that there was no significant difference in the enamel and dentine mineral densities between the control and experimental diabetes groups (Fig. 12). However, the type 1 diabetes group showed a significant decrease in the thickness of enamel and dentine surfaces when compared to the control group (Fig. 13) [79].

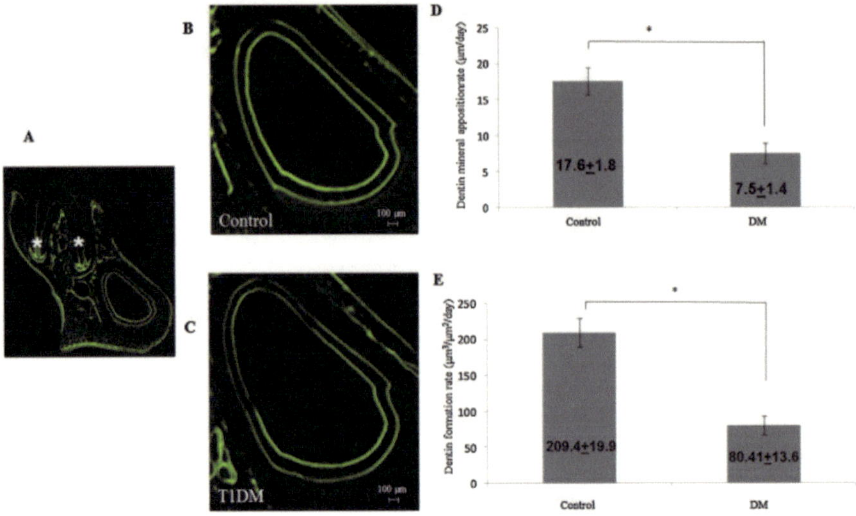

Figure 11. (A) Frontal section of the lower right mandible. *The lower first molar two roots that were considered the landmark for cutting all samples. (B, C) Frontal sections of the rat incisor mandibular first molar area. (B) Control; (C) T1DM. Fluorescent labelling indicates the new dentine formation. (D) The mineral apposition rate (MAR) of the dentine mandibular incisor for the control group and the T1DM group. The data are expressed as means ± SD. $n = 10$ for each group. Significant difference from controls, with $^*P < 0.05$. (E) The dentine formation rate (DFR) of the dentine mandibular incisor for the control group and the DM group. The data are expressed as means ± S.D. $n = 10$ for each group. Significant difference from controls, with $^*P < 0.05$).

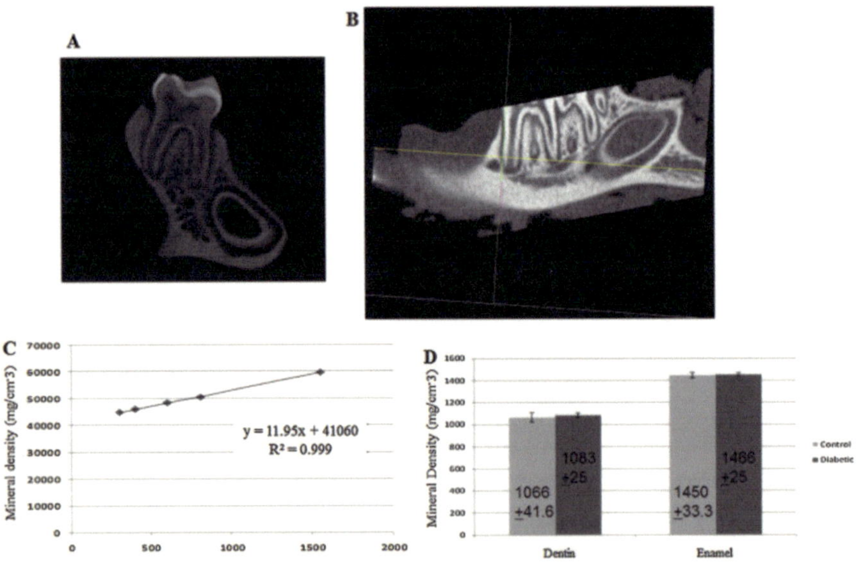

Figure 12. (A) Representative 3D reconstruction of the left mandible imaged by micro-CT. (B) The left mandible with the vertical reference line extending parallel to the mesial surface of the first molar. (C) Mineral density calibration curve based on the gray scale values obtained from the mineral reference phantoms (linear regression, R2 > 0.99). (D) Graph showing that there is no significant difference in the incisor enamel and dentine mineral densities between the control and T1DM groups.

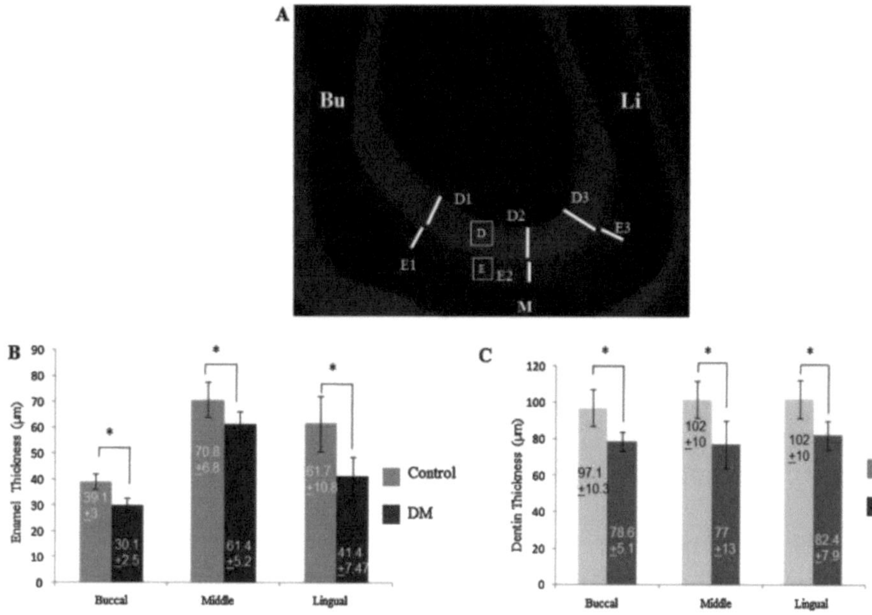

Figure 13. (A) The micro-CT oriented image of the rat mandibular incisor showing the three zones (E1–E3) selected for evaluation of enamel thickness and the three zones (D1–D3) selected for evaluation of dentine thickness. B-buccal; M-middle; Li-lingual. (B) The T1DM group shows a significant decrease in the thickness of enamel surface when compared to control group in the three different zones. (C) The T1DM group shows a significant decrease in the thickness of dentine surface when compared to control group in the three different zones ($P < 0.05$).

3.10. Suggested mechanism for the effect of diabetic condition on craniofacial complex

Growth of the craniofacial or maxillofacial complex is regulated by genetic and environmental factors [57]. For normal growth and morphogenesis of the cranial and maxillofacial complex, a proper regulation by hormones, nutrients, mechanical forces, and various general and local growth factor is essential. Type 1 diabetes causes a deteriorating growth and metabolic disorder of bone in both humans and experimental animals [58]. Since studies in humans are generally limited by small sample size, cross-sectional designs, uncontrolled variables, and often retrospective natures; it often performed more rigorous analyses using animal models [56]. We have observed the growth of the rat from 3 weeks of age to 7 weeks of age in our study. According to the previous craniofacial growth studies, this period corresponds to the initial stage of growth in humans [80, 81]. Consequently, STZ-induced DM models in our study were used to investigate the effects of type 1 diabetes on the development of craniofacial complex. These STZ-induced DM rats showed a significant reduction in the growth of a large portion of the unit of craniofacial hard tissues compared with control rats, but regarding the rest of the craniofacial skeletal units (sphenoid bone length, posterior neurocranium height, anterior corpus length, bigonial width, and palatal width), no significant difference were observed between the control and the STZ-induced DM groups. In general, craniofacial skeletal growth was significantly lower in STZ-induced DM group compared to controls in all three dimensions. The previous study investigated the DM effect exclusively on the growth of the mandible and suggested that the diabetic condition had a differential effect on the osseous components and/or its associated non-skeletal tissues. They discussed that disharmony of the mandibular growth was due to the condition of the DM, such as renal failure, anemia, body weight change, or alteration in the food-intake qualities [58]. Thus, we hypothesize that the deficiency in the craniofacial growth in our experiment might be due to the diabetic condition in the DM group as it has been reported that specific changes in bone metabolism are associated with DM. In addition, some of the pathogenic potential, insulinopenia, microvascular bone, dysregulation of mineral metabolism, changes in local factors that regulate bone remodeling, and even an intrinsic disorder related to type 1 diabetes, have been proposed [82, 83]. It is thought that the aforementioned deficiency of the insulin associated with type 1 diabetes may have a direct effect on bone metabolism. It was reported that normal insulin levels exert a direct anabolic effect on bone cells [82]. Multiple osteoblast-like cell lines, expressing the insulin receptor on the cell surface, have a high capacity for insulin binding [84]. Moreover, osteoclast are known to reduce bone resorption in response to insulin stimulation [85]. These findings support the view that insulin in bone can act directly against osteoblasts in combination with the inhibition of osteoclasts [60, 85], and this mechanism of action can be used to explain the delay in the craniofacial growth in STZ-DM. Diabetes has a detrimental effect on osseous turnover due to decreased both osteoblast and osteoclast activities and numbers and, a lower percentage of osteoid surface and osteocalcin synthesis, as well as increased time for mineralization of osteoid [82]. In a separate stage in matrix-induced endochondral bone formation, the influence of diabetes was reported to have a significant impact on the biomechanical behavior of bone. In addition, chondrogenesis and calcification of bone were reduced by 50% in diabetic animals [86]. This was also consistent with our findings that showed a significant reduction in the craniofacial linear measurements of the DM group. In addition, insulin can exert synergistic effects with other anabolic agents on bone, such as parathyroid hormone (PTH) [60, 85]. Type 1 diabetes animal models frequently show the alteration in bone turnover, retarded growth, increased concentration of PTH, and reduced concentration of 1,25-dihydroxyvitamin D [82, 87]. The effects of PTH on the bones are rather complex; PTH stimulates resorption or bone formation depending on the concentration used, the duration of the exhibition, and the administration method [82, 86, 87, 88]. Moreover, 1,25-dihydroxivitamin D, like PTH, belongs to the most important group of bone regulatory hormones. It regulates osteoclastic differentiation from hematopoietic mononuclear cells, and osteoblastic functions and activity [82, 89].

Moreover, insulin may indirectly regulate the increase in the concentration of growth hormone (GH) in serum concentration by direct regulation of the hepatic growth hormone receptor. That would result in abnormalities in the insulin growth factor-1 (IGF-1) in T1DM [90] which consequently might have led to the retarded growth in uncontrolled DM, in our study. In the present study, the mineral appositional rates and bone formation rate in DM group were significantly lower in the most area of periosteal surface in mandible as compared to the control group. These results are in agreement with the previous studies that reported diminished lamellar bone formation in DM rats' femur and may suggesting the putative association between the DM condition and the decreased number and function of osteoblasts [61]. The alveolar crest region was the only region that did not show a significant difference in the mineral apposition rate and the bone formation rate parameters between healthy and DM groups; this may be attributed to the unique nature of this region exhibiting a highly intensive bone remodeling process especially during the teeth eruption that decreases toward the base of the socket [77]. A significant decrease in bone volume fraction, trabecular thickness, and trabecular numbers was confirmed by micro-CT analysis in DM rats. DM rats also showed a significant increase in the trabecular separation and the trabecular space when compared with the control group. This finding indicated the deterioration of the bone quality in the DM group. These observations are in agreement with other works suggesting that the glycemic levels play an important role in modulating the trabecular architecture especially in mandibular bone [60]. In this context, these results may describe a state of osteopenia in experimental diabetic rats, which might be caused by an imbalance between bone formation and resorption. A histometric evaluation of bone resorption was performed by counting the number of osteoclast cells on the distal surface of the alveolar bone adjacent to the mesio-buccal root of the second molar. These evaluations revealed that the number of osteoclasts was significantly lower in the DM rats than in the controls, in line with the previous studies on DM rats' mandible and long bones [58]. These studies confirm that the decreased rate of bone turnover may be associated with the DM condition. This worsening effect of the structure and dynamic bone formation on mandible might be due to a number of pathogenic potentials such as insulinopenia, bone microangiopathy, impaired regulation of mineral metabolism, alteration in local factors that regulate bone remodeling [57, 83]. However, the adverse effects observed may not be associated with the significant loss of rats' weights observed in the diabetic group starting from day 14 because previous research [57, 60] showed that the mandibular growth was not affected in normal rats supplied with restricted diet and having same pattern of weight loss resembling weight loss pattern observed in DM rats.

3.11. Expected mechanism of type 1 diabetes detrimental effects on tooth

Many investigations focused on the various detrimental effects exerted by the type 1 diabetes on different body organs; however, less attention was paid to the effect of such condition on teeth. A previous study suggested that the diabetic condition may exert detrimental effects on enamel formation [91]. However, that study was conducted on an extremely small sample size of different types of rodents suffering from diabetic conditions that were either genetically induced or drug induced and did not include a proper number of control rats. Thus, it was of an extreme importance to study the detrimental effect of diabetes on tooth structure formation using enough number of experimental animals and to use accurate methods of measurements as those adopted in the our studies. The null hypotheses tested in our previous study were partly accepted because the type 1 diabetes condition adversely affected the enamel and dentine thickness, and the dentine mineral apposition and dentine formation rates; however, there was no significant effect of the type 1 diabetes condition on the enamel and dentine mineral densities.

We have demonstrated that the type 1 diabetes condition induced detrimental changes on the thickness of enamel and dentine. Thus, it could be speculated that the metabolic functions of the ameloblasts and the odontoblasts may be hindered by the elevated blood glucose level associated with the type 1 diabetes condition. It was previously suggested that the type 1 diabetes condition affect ameloblasts and odontoblasts by a mechanism similar to the well-documented mechanism exerted by the type 1 diabetes condition on osteoblasts bone-forming cells due to the similarities between the process of dentine, enamel, and bone development [92]. Moreover, several genetic disorders were found to affect both the osteoblasts and odontoblasts and thus affecting the mineralization process of bone and dentine, respectively [92]. However, in contrast to bone, dentine and enamel do not remodel and are not involved in the regulation of the calcium and phosphate metabolism [93].

It was previously demonstrated that a glucose concentration similar to those observed in poorly controlled diabetic patients inhibited the osteoblast cells from depositing calcium during the mineralization process of the bone matrix [94]. One can speculate that a similar inhibitory effect was exhibited in the current study by the high glucose level on the activities of the odontoblasts and ameloblasts during the enamel and dentine formation. This inhibitory effect of increased glucose level on ameloblasts and odontoblasts was suggested by a previous study that showed that the total calcium content in rat teeth suffering from type 1 diabetes was significantly lower than those of their controls [95]. Another study reported a significant decrease in cultured pulp cells ability to proliferate and decreased mineralized nodule formation upon exposure to high levels of glucose [96]. Another mechanism that might explain the negative effects exerted by the type 1 diabetes condition on odontoblasts and ameloblasts activities may be attributed to the increase in blood glucose level that interferes with the maturation and the proper mineralization of the dentine collagen matrix during the dentine development stages [97]. Previous research work showed that the histological features of the ameloblast and its function might be affected by the increased glucose level associated with the type 1 diabetes condition [98]. Moreover, several clinical observations showed that enamel susceptibility to caries and the incidence of enamel hypoplasia increased in type 1 diabetes patients [99]. Furthermore, it was previously suggested that type 1 diabetes condition may exert a generalized decrease in the metabolic activities of bone cells. All of the aforementioned findings may suggest that the observed harmful effects exerted by the type 1 diabetes condition on enamel and dentine in this study may be a part of a generalized detrimental effect exerted by the diabetic condition on osteoblasts, odontoblasts, and ameloblasts.

4. Conclusion

It is obvious that type 1 diabetes condition significantly affects craniofacial growth, bone formation mechanism, and the quality of the bone formed, which may alter many aspects of planning and treatment of orthodontic patients affected by this globally increasing hormonal disturbance. Moreover, type 1 diabetes condition impairs the proper tooth development and alters the oral environment rendering teeth more susceptible to dental caries. There should be a new strategy for treating orthodontic patients suffering from metabolic disorders specially those disorders having direct and indirect effects on bone growth as the diabetic condition. The orthodontic craniofacial linear measurements were significantly decreased in the type 1 diabetes cases when compared to normal cases. Moreover, greater risks of developing dental caries and possible tooth loss are associated with patients suffering from type 1 diabetes; these risks may complicate the outcome of orthodontic treatment which is associated with less ability of orthodontic patients to implement proper oral hygiene measures due to increased areas of bacterial biofilm formation around orthodontic brackets. These comprehensive studies carried out on bone and craniofacial growth suggest that planning the treatment in craniofacial region for patients affected with hormonal disorders is more complex procedure than the treatment of normal patients. Up-to-date data also suggest that it is of prime importance to keep close attention to the general systemic condition of these patients and administer the proper hormonal therapy for these patients when needed to avoid any detrimental effects on bone resulting from any hormonal imbalance. Moreover, the results of tooth analysis in experimental type 1 diabetes model showed that the type 1 diabetes condition suppressed the enamel and dentine formation; however, the enamel and dentine densities were not affected. This indicates that diabetic patients may be more susceptible to dental caries and teeth size discrepancies. Type 1 diabetes patients' dental problems should be handled carefully, and their diabetic condition monitoring is of prime importance, especially during early stage of tooth development.

Author details

Ippei Watari[1*], Mona Aly Abbassy[2,3], Katarzyna Anna Podyma-Inoue[4] and Takashi Ono[1]

*Address all correspondence to: ippeiwatari@gmail.com

1 Orthodontic Science, Department of Orofacial Development and Function, Division of Oral Health Science, Graduate School of Medical and Dental Science, Tokyo Medical and Dental University (TMDU), Tokyo, Japan

2 Department of Orthodontics, Faculty of Dentistry, King Abdulaziz University, Jeddah, Saudi Arabia

3 Alexandria University, Alexandria, Egypt

4 Section of Biochemistry, Department of Bio-Matrix, Graduate School of Medical and Dental Science, Tokyo Medical and Dental University (TMDU), Tokyo, Japan

References

[1] Harjutsalo, V., Sjoberg, L., & Tuomilehto, J. (2008). Time trends in the incidence of type 1 diabetes in Finnish Children: a cohort study. *Lancet*, 371 (9626), 1777–1782.

[2] Onkamo, P., Vaananen, S., Karvonen, M., & Tuomilehto, J. (1999). Worldwide increase in incidence of type 1 diabetes—the analysis of the data on published incidence trends. *Diabetologia*, 42 (12), 1395–1403.

[3] WURODIAB ACE Study Group. (2000). Variation and trends in incidence of childhood diabetes in Surope. *Lancet*, 355, 873–876.

[4] Guariguata, L. (2011). Estimating the worldwide burden of type 1 diabetes. *Diabetes Voice*, 56(2), 6–8.

[5] Zhukouskaya V, Eller-Vainicher C, Shepelkevich AP, Dydyshko Y, Cairoli E, Chiodini I. (2015) Bone health in type 1 diabetes: focus on evaluation and treatment in clinical practice. Journal of Endocrinological Investigation 38(9) 941-950.

[6] Janghormani, M., van Dam, R. M., Willett W. C., & Hu, F. B. (2007). Systemic review of type 1 and type 2 diabetes mellitus and risk of fracture. *American Journal Epidemiology*, 166, 495–505.

[7] Vestergaard, P., (2007). Discrepancies in bone mineral density and fracture risk in patients with type 1 and type 2 diabetes—a metanalysis. *Osteoporosis International*, 18, 427–444.

[8] Hamada, Y., Kitazawa, S., Kitazawa, R., Fujii, H., Kasuga, M., & Fukagawa, M. (2007). Histomorphometric analysis of diabetic osteopenia in streptozotocin-induced diabetic mice: a possible role of oxidative stress. *Bone*, 40(5), 1408–1418.

[9] Lu, H., Kraut D., Gerstenfeld, L. C., & Graves, D. T. (2003). Diabetes interferes with the bone formation by affecting the expression of transcription factors that regulate osteoblast differentiation. *Endocrinology*, 144(1), 346–352.

[10] Reddy, G. K., Stehno-Bittel, L., Hamade, S., & Enwemeka, C. S. (2001). The biomechanical integrity of bone in experimental diabetes. *Diabetes Research Clinical Practice*, 54(1), 1–8.

[11] Ogata, N., Chikazu, D., Kubota, N., Terauchi, Y., Tobe, K., Azuma, Y., Ohta, T., Kadowaki, T., Nakamura, K., & Kawaguchi, H. (2000). Insulin receptor substrate-1 in osteoblast is indispensable for maintaining bone turnover. *Journal of Clinical Investigation*, 105 (7), 935–943.

[12] Albright, F., & Reifestein, E. C. (1948). Bone development in diabetic children: a roentgen study. *The American Journal of the Medical Sciences*, 174, 313–319.

[13] Levin, M. E., Boisseau, V. C., & Avioli, L. V. (1976). Effects of diabetes mellitus on bone mass in juvenile and adult onset diabetes. *The New England Journal of Medicine*, 294(5), 241–245.

[14] Munoz-Torres, M., Jodar, E., Escobar-Jimenez, F., López-Ibarra, P. J., & Luna, J. D. (1996). Bone mineral density measured by dual X-ray absorptiometry in Spanish patients with insulin-dependent diabetes mellitus. *Calcified Tissue International*, 58 (5), 316–319.

[15] Miazgowski, T., & Czekalski, S. (1998). A 2-year follow-up study on bone mineral density and markers of bone turnover in patients with long-standing insulin-dependent diabetes mellitus. *Osteoporosis International,* 8(5), 399–403.

[16] Jehle, P. M., Jehle, E. R., Mohan, S., & Böhm, B. O. (1998). Serum levels of insulin-like growth factor system components and relationship to bone metabolism in type 1 and type 2 diabetes mellitus patients. *Journal of Endocrinology,* 159(2), 297–306.

[17] Tuominen, J. T., Impivaara, O., Puukka, P., & Rönnemaa, T. (1999). Bone mineral density in patients with type 1 and type 2 diabetes. *Diabetes Care,* 22(7), 1196–200.

[18] Gallacher, S. J., Fenner, J. A., Fischer, B. M., Quin, J. D., Fraser, W. D., Logue, F. C., Cowan, R. A., Boyle, I. T., & MacCuish, A. C. (1993). An evaluation of bone density and turnover in premenopausal women with type 1 diabetes mellitus. *Diabetic Medicine,* 10(2), 129–133.

[19] Weber, G., Beccaria, L., deAngelis, M., Mora, S., Galli, L., Cazzuffi, M., A., Turba, F., Frisone, F., Guarneri, M., P., & Chiumello, G. (1990). Bone mass in young patients with type 1 diabetes. *Bone and Mineral,* 8(1), 23–30.

[20] Pascual, J., Argente, J., & Lopezetal M. B. (1998). Bone mineral density in children and adolescents with diabetes mellitus type 1 of recent onset. *Calcified Tissue International,* 62(1), 31–35.

[21] Salvatoni, A., Mancassola, G., Biasoli, R., Cardani, R., Salvatore, S., Broggini, M., & Nespoli, L. (2004). Bone mineral density in diabetic children and adolescents: a follow-up study. *Bone,* 34(5), 900–904.

[22] Brandao, F. R., Vicente, E. J., Daltro, C. H., Sacramento, M., Moreira, A., & Adan, L. (2007). Bone metabolism is linked to disease duration and metabolic control in type 1 diabetes mellitus. *Diabetes Research and Clinical Practice,* 78(3), 334–339.

[23] Liu, E. Y., Wactawski-Wende, J., Donahue, R. P., Dmochowski, J., Hovey, K. M., & Quattrin T. (2003). Does low bone mineral density start in post-teenage years in women with type 1 diabetes? *Diabetes Care,* 26(8), 2365–2369.

[24] Mastrandrea, L. D., Wactawski-Wende, J., Donahue, R. P., Hovey, K. M., Clark, A., & Quattrin, T. (2008). Young women with type 1 diabetes have lower bone mineral density that persists over time. *Diabetes Care,* 31(9), 1729–1735.

[25] Bechtold, S., Dirlenbach, I., Raile, K., Noelle, V., Bonfig, W., & Schwarz, H. P. (2006). Early manifestation of type 1 diabetes in children is a risk factor for changed bone geometry: data using peripheral quantitative computed tomography. *Pediatrics,* 118(3), e627–e634.

[26] Maggio, A. B. R., Ferrari, S., & Kraenzlinetal, M. (2010). Decreased bone turnover in children and adolescents with well controlled type 1 diabetes. *Journal of Pediatric Endocrinology and Metabolism,* 23(7), 697–707.

[27] Gunczler, P., Lanes, R., Paz-Martinez, V., Martins, R., Esaa, S., Colmenares, V., & Weisinger, J., R. (1998). Decreased lumbar spine bone mass and low bone turnover in children and adolescents with insulin dependent diabetes mellitus followed longitudinally. *Journal of Pediatric Endocrinology and Metabolism*, 11(3), 413–419.

[28] Valerio, G., del Puente, A., Esposito-del Puente, A., Buono, P., Mozzillo, E., & Franzese, A. (2002). The lumbar bone mineral density is affected by long-term poor metabolic control in adolescents with type1 diabetes mellitus. *Hormone Research*, 58(6), 266–272.

[29] Heilman, K., Zilmer, M., Zilmer, K., & Tillmann, V. (2009). Lower bone mineral density in children with type 1 diabetes is associated with poor glycemic control and higher serum ICAM1 and urinary isoprostane levels. *Journal of Bone and Mineral Metabolism*, 27(5), 598–604.

[30] L′eger, J., Marinovic, D., Alberti, C., Dorgeret, S., Chevenne, D., Marchal, C. L., Tubiana-Rufi, N., Sebag, G., & Czernichow, P. (2006). Lower bone mineral content in children with type 1 diabetes mellitus is linked to female sex, low insulin-like growth factor type I levels, and high insulin requirement. *Journal of Clinical Endocrinology and Metabolism*, 91(10), 3947–3953.

[31] Saha, M. T. Sievänen, H., Salo, M., K. Tulokas, S., & Saha, H. H. (2009). Bone mass and structure in adolescents with type 1 diabetes compared to healthy peers. *Osteoporosis International*, 20(8), 1401–1406.

[32] Heap, J., Murray, M. A., Miller, S. C., Jalili, T., & Moyer Mileur, L. J. (2004). Alterations in bone characteristics associated with glycemic control in adolescents with type 1 diabetes mellitus. *Journal of Pediatrics*, 144(1), 56–62.

[33] Hamed, E. A., Abu Faddan, N. H., Adb Elhafeez, H. A., & Sayed, D. (2011). Parathormone—25(OH)-vitamin D axis and bone status in children and adolescents with type1 diabetes mellitus. *Pediatric Diabetes*, 12(6), 536–546.

[34] Liu, E. Y., Wactawski-Wende, J., Donahue, R. P., Dmochowski, J., Hovey, K. M., & Quattrin, T. (2003). Does low bone mineral density start in post-teenage years in women with type 1 diabetes? *Diabetes Care*, 26(8), 2365–2389.

[35] Mastrandrea, L. D., Wactawski-Wenda, J., Donahue, R. P., Hovey, K. M., Clark, A., & Quattrin, T. (2008). Young women with type 1 diabetes have lower bone mineral density that persists over time. *Diabetes Care*, 31(9), 1729–1735.

[36] Kemink, S. A. G., Hermus, A. R. M. M., Swinkels, L. M. J. W., Lutterman, J. A., & Smals, A. G. H. (2000). Osteopenia in insulin-dependent diabetes mellitus: prevalence and aspects of pathophysiology. *Journal of Endocrinology Investigation*, 23(5), 295–303.

[37] Rozasilla, A., Nolla, J. M., Montana, E., Fiter, J., Gomez-Vaquero, C., Soler, J., & Roig-Escofet, D. (2000). Bone mineral density in patients with type 1 diabetes mellitus. *Joint Bone Spine*, 67(3), 215–218.

[38] Hadjidakis, D. J., Raptis, A. E., Sfakianakis, M., Mylonakis, A., & Raptis, S. A. (2006). Bone mineral density of both genders in type 1 diabetes according to bone composition. *Journal of Diabetes and its Complications*, 20(5), 302–307.

[39] Danielson, K. K., Elliott, M. E., Lecaire, T., Binkley, N., & Palta, M. (2009). Poor glycemic control is associated with low BMD detected in premenopausal women with type 1 diabetes. *Osteoporosis International*, 20(6), 923–933.

[40] Alexopoulou, O., Jamart, J., Devogelaer, J. P., Brichard, S. de Nayer, P., & Buyysschaert, M. (2006). Bone density and markers of bone remodeling in type 1 male diabetic patients. *Diabetes and Metabolism*, 32(5), 453–458.

[41] Hampson, G., Evans, C., Petttit, R. J., Evans, W. D., Woodhead, S. J., Peters, J. R., & Ralston, S. H. (1998). Bone mineral density, collagen type 1 alpha 1 genotypes and bone turnover in premenopausal women with diabetes mellitus. *Diabetologia*, 41(11), 1314–1320.

[42] Ingberg, C. M., Palmer, M., Aman, J., Arvidsson, B., Schvarcz, E., & Berne, C. (2004). Body composition and bone mineral density in long-standing type 1 diabetes. *Journal of International Medicine*, 255(3), 392–398.

[43] Bridges, M. J., Moochhala, S. H., Barbour, J., & Kelly, C. A. (2005). Influence of diabetes on peripheral bone mineral density in men: a controlled study. *Acta Diabetologica*, 42(2), 82–86.

[44] Vestergaard, P. (2007). Discrepancies in bone mineral density and fracture risk in patients with type 1 and type 2 diabetes—a meta-analysis. *Osteoporosis International*, 18(4), 427–444.

[45] Zhukouskaya V. V., Eller-Vainicher C., Vadzianava V. V., Shepelkevich A. P., Zhurava I. V., Korolenko G. G., Salko O. B., Cairoli E., Beck-Peccoz P., Chiodini I. (2013) Prevalence of morphometric vertebral fractures in patients with type 1 diabetes. Diabetes Care, 36(6):1635-40.

[46] Inoue, Y., Hisa, I., Seino, S., & Kaji, H. (2010). Alendronate induces mineralization in mouse osteoblastic MC3T3-E1 cells: regulation of mineralization-related genes. *Experimental Clinical Endocrinology and Diabetes*, 118(10), 719–723.

[47] Aoyama, E., Watari, I., Podyma-Inoue, K. A., Yanagishita, M., & Ono, T. (2014). Expression of glucagon-like peptide-1 receptor and glucose-dependent insulinotropic polypeptide receptor is regulated by the glucose concentration in mouse osteoblastic MC3T3-E1 cells. *International Journal of Molecular Medicine*, 34(2), 475–478.

[48] Baggio, L. L., & Drucker, D. J. (2007). Biology of incretins: GLP-1 and GIP. *Gastroenterology*, 132(6), 2131–2157.

[49] Yamada, C., Yamada, Y., Tsukiyama, K., Yamada, K., Udagawa, N., Takahashi, N., Tanaka, K., Drucker, D. J., Seino, Y., & Inagaki, N. (2008). The murine glucagon-like peptide-1 receptor is essential for control of bone resorption. *Endocrinology*, 149(2), 574–579.

[50] Driessen, J. H., van Onzenoort, H. A., Henry, R. M., Lalmohamed, A., van den Bergh, J. P., Neef, C., Leufkens, H. G., & de Vries, F. (2014). Use of dipeptidyl peptidase-4 inhibitors for type 2 diabetes mellitus and risk of fracture. *Bone*, 68, 124–130.

[51] Bensch, L., Braem, M., Van Acker, K., & Willems, G. (2003). Orthodontic treatment considerations in patients with diabetes mellitus. *American Journal of Orthodontics and Dentofacial Orthopedics*, 123(1), 74–78.

[52] Giglio, M. J., & Lama, M. A. (2001). Effect of experimental diabetes on mandible growth in rats. *European Journal of Oral Sciences*, 109(3), 193–197.

[53] Salzmann, J. A. (1979). Practice of orthodontics under public health guidance. *American Journal of Orthodontics*, 76(1), 103–104.

[54] Kumar, P., & Clark, M. (2009). Kumar and Clark's Clinical Medicine (7th edition), Elsevier.

[55] El-Bialy, T., Aboul-Azm, S. F., & El-Sakhawy, M. (2000). Study of craniofacial morphology and skeletal maturation in juvenile diabetics (type I). *American Journal of Orthodontics and Dentofacial Orthopedics*, 118(2), 189–195.

[56] Roe, T. F., Mora, S., Costen, G., Kaufman, F., Carlson, M., & Gilsanz, V. (1991). Vertebral bone density in insulin-dependent diabetic children. *Metabolism*, 40(9), 967–971.

[57] Abbassy, M. A., Watari, I., & Soma, K. (2008). Effect of experimental diabetes on craniofacial growth in rats. *Archives of Oral Biology*, 53(9), 819–825.

[58] Hough, S., Avioli, L. V., Bergfeld, M. A., Fallon, M. D., Slatopolsky, E., & Teitelbaum, S. L. (1981). Correction of abnormal bone and mineral metabolism in chronic streptozotocin-induced diabetes mellitus in the rat by insulin therapy. *Endocrinology*, 108(6), 2228–2234.

[59] Tein, MS, Breen, S. A., Loveday, B. E., Devlin, H., Balment, R. J., Boyd, R. D., Sibley CP, Garland HO.. (1998). Bone mineral density and composition in rat pregnancy: effects of streptozotocin-induced diabetes mellitus and insulin replacement. *Experimental Physiology*, 83(2), 165–174.

[60] Thrailkill, K. M., Liu, L., Wahl, E. C., Bunn, R. C., Perrien, D. S., Cockrell, G. E., Skinner RA, Hogue WR, Carver AA, Fowlkes JL, Aronson J, Lumpkin CK Jr. (2005). Bone formation is impaired in a model of type 1 diabetes. *Diabetes*, 54(10), 2875–2881.

[61] Follak, N., Kloting, I., Wolf, E., & Merk, H. (2004). Histomorphometric evaluation of the influence of the diabetic metabolic state on bone defect healing depending on the defect size in spontaneously diabetic BB/OK rats. *Bone*, 35(1), 144–152.

[62] Alkan, A., Erdem, E., Gunhan, O., & Karasu, C. (2002). Histomorphometric evaluation of the effect of doxycycline on the healing of bone defects in experimental diabetes mellitus: a pilot study. *Journal of Oral and Maxillofacial Surgery*, 60(8), 898–904.

[63] Mc Cracken-Wesson, M. S., Aponte, R., Chavali, R., & Lemons, J. E. (2006). Bone associated with implants in diabetic and insulin-treated rats. *Clinical Oral Implants Research*, 17(5), 495–500.

[64] Abdus, Salam. M., Matsumoto, N., Matin, K., Tsuha, Y., Nakao, R., Hanada, N., & Senpuku, H. (2004). Establishment of an animal model using recombinant NOD.B10.D2 mice to study initial adhesion of oral streptococci. *Clinical and Diagnostic Laboratory Immunology*, 11(2), 379–386.

[65] Matin, K., Salam, M. A., Akhter, J., Hanada, N., & Senpuku, H. (2002). Role of stromal-cell derived factor-1 in the development of autoimmune diseases in non-obese diabetic mice. *Immunology*, 107(2), 222–232.

[66] Chidiac, J. J., Shofer, F. S., Al-Kutoub, A., Laster, L. L., & Ghafari, J. (2002). Comparison of CT scanograms and cephalometric radiographs in craniofacial imaging. *Orthodontics and Craniofacial Research*, 5(2), 104–113.

[67] Vande Berg, J. R., Buschang, P. H., & Hinton, R. J. (2004). Absolute and relative growth of the rat craniofacial skeleton. *Archives of Oral Biology*, 49(6), 477–484.

[68] Engstrom, C., Jennings, J., Lundy, M., & Baylink, D. J. (1988). Effect of bone matrix-derived growth factors on skull and tibia in the growing rat. *Journal of Oral Pathology*, 17(7), 334–340.

[69] Kiliaridis, S. E. C., & Thilander, B. (1985). The relationship between masticatory function and craniofacial morphology. I. A cephalometric longitudinal analysis in the growing rat fed a soft diet. *European Journal of Orthodontics*, 7, 273–283.

[70] Vandeberg, J. R., Buschang, P. H., & Hinton, R. J. (2004). Craniofacial growth in growth hormone-deficient rats. The anatomical record. Part A. *Discoveries in Molecular, Cellular and Evolutionary Biology*, 278(2), 561–570.

[71] Stuart, A., & Smith, D. (1992). Use of the fluorochromes xylenol orange, calcein green, and tetracycline to document bone deposition and remodeling in healing fractures in chickens. *Avian Diseases*, 36 (2), 447–449.

[72] Abbassy, M. A., Watari, I., & Soma, K. (2010). The effect of diabetes mellitus on rat mandibular bone formation and microarchitecture. *European Journal of Oral Sciences*, 118(4), 364–369.

[73] Shimomoto, Y., Chung, C. J., Iwasaki-Hayashi, Y., Muramoto, T., & Soma, K. (2007). Effects of occlusal stimuli on alveolar/jaw bone formation. *Journal of Dental Research*, 86(1), 47–51.

[74] Parfitt, A. M. (1988). Bone histomorphometry: standardization of nomenclature, symbols and units (summary of proposed system). *Bone*, 9(1), 67–69.

[75] Keshawarz, N. M., & Recker, R. R. (1986). The label escape error: comparison of measured and theoretical fraction of total bone-trabecular surface covered by single label in normals and patients with osteoporosis. *Bone*, 7(2), 83–87.

[76] Sheng, M. H., Baylink, D. J., Beamer, W. G., Donahue, L. R., Rosen, C. J., Lau, K. H., Wergedal JE. (1999). Histomorphometric studies show that bone formation and bone mineral apposition rates are greater in C3H/HeJ (high-density) than C57BL/6J (low-density) mice during growth. *Bone*, 25(4), 421–429.

[77] Gerlach, R. F., Toledo, D. B., Fonseca, R. B., Novaes, P. D., Line, S. R., & Merzel, J. (2002). Alveolar bone remodelling pattern of the rat incisor under different functional conditions as shown by minocycline administration. *Archives of Oral Biology*, 47(3), 203–209.

[78] Siudikiene, J., Machiulskiene, V., Nyvad, B., Tenovuo, J., & Nedzelskiene, I. (2006). Dental caries and salivary status in children with type 1 diabetes mellitus, related to the metabolic control of the disease. *European Journal of Oral Sciences*, 114(1), 8–14.

[79] Abbassy, M. A., Watari, I., Barkry, A. S., Hamba, H., Hassan, A. H., Tagami, T., & Ono, T. (2015). Diabetes detrimental effects on enamel and dentin formation. *Journal of Dentistry*, 43(5), 589–596.

[80] Losken, A., Mooney, M. P., & Siegel, M. I. (1994). Comparative cephalometric study of nasal cavity growth patterns in seven animal models. *Cleft Palate Craniofacial Journal*, 31(1), 17–23.

[81] Siegel, M. I., & Mooney, M. P. (1990). Appropriate animal models for craniofacial biology. *Cleft Palate Journal*, 27(1), 18–25.

[82] Duarte, V. M., Ramos, A. M., Rezende, L. A., Macedo, U. B., Brandao-Neto, J., Almeida, M. G., & Rezende, A. A. (2005). Osteopenia: a bone disorder associated with diabetes mellitus. *Journal of Bone and Mineral Metabolism*, 23(1), 58–68.

[83] Ward, D. T., Yau, S. K., Mee, A. P., Mawer, E. B., Miller, CA, Garland, H. O., et al. (2001). Functional, molecular, and biochemical characterization of streptozotocin-induced diabetes. *Journal of the American Society of Nephrology*, 12(4), 779–790.

[84] Pun, K. K., Lau, P., & Ho, P. W. (1989). The characterization, regulation, and function of insulin receptors on osteoblast-like clonal osteosarcoma cell line. *Journal of Bone and Mineral Research*, 4(6), 853–862.

[85] Thomas, D. M., Udagawa, N., Hards, D. K., Quinn, J. M., Moseley, J. M., Findlay, D. M., Best JD. (1998). Insulin receptor expression in primary and cultured osteoclast-like cells. *Bone*, 23(3), 181–186

[86] Reddy, G. K., Stehno-Bittel, L., Hamade, S., & Enwemeka, C. S. (2001). The biomechanical integrity of bone in experimental diabetes. *Diabetes Research and Clinical Practice*, 54(1), 1–8.

[87] Tsuchida, T., Sato, K., Miyakoshi, N., Abe, T., Kudo, T., Tamura, Y., Kasukawa Y, Suzuki K. (2000). Histomorphometric evaluation of the recovering effect of human parathyroid hormone (1–34) on bone structure and turnover in streptozotocin-induced diabetic rats. *Calcified Tissue International*, 66(3), 229–233.

[88] Toromanoff, A., Ammann, P., Mosekilde, L., Thomsen, J. S., & Riond, J. L. (1997). Parathyroid hormone increases bone formation and improves mineral balance in vitamin D-deficient female rats. *Endocrinology*, 138(6), 2449–2457.

[89] Collins, D., Jasani, C., Fogelman, I., & Swaminathan, R. (1998). Vitamin D and bone mineral density. *Osteoporosis International*, 8(2), 110–114.

[90] Chiarelli, F., Giannini, C., & Mohn, A. (2004). Growth, growth factors and diabetes. *European Journal of Endocrinology*, 151(3), U109–U117.

[91] Atar, M., Atar-Zwillenberg, D. R., Verry, P., & Spornitz, U. M. (2004). Defective enamel ultrastructure in diabetic rodents. *International Journal of Paediatric Dentistry*, 14, 301–307.

[92] Opsahl Vital, S., Gaucher, C., Bardet, C., Rowe, P. S., George, A., Linglart, A., & Chaussain, C. (2012). Tooth dentin defects reflect genetic disorders affecting bone mineralization. *Bone*, 50(4), 989–997.

[93] Chen, S., Rani, S., Wu, Y., Unterbrink, A., Gu, T. T., Gluhak-Heinrich, J, Chuang, H. H., & Macdougall, M. (2005). Differential regulation of dentin sialophosphoprotein expression by Runx2 during odontoblast cytodifferentiation. *The Journal of Biological Chemistry*, 280(33), 29717–29727.

[94] Balint, E., Szabo, P., Marshall, C. F., & Sprague, S. M. (2001). Glucose-induced inhibition of in vitro bone mineralization. *Bone*, 28 (1), 21–28.

[95] Gutowska, I., Baranowska-Bosiacka, I., Rybicka, M., Nocen, I., Dudzinska, W., Marchlewicz, M., Wiszniewska, B., & Chlubek, D. (2011). Changes in the concentration of microelements in the teeth of rats in the final stage of type 1 diabetes, with an absolute lack of insulin. *Biology of Trace Element Research*, 139(3), 332–340.

[96] Yeh, C. K., Harris, S. E., Mohan, S., Horn, D., Fajardo, R., Chun, Y. H., Jorgensen, J., Macdougall, M., & Abboud-Werner, S. (2012). Hyperglycemia and xerostomia are key determinants of tooth decay in type 1 diabetic mice. *Laboratory Investigation*, 92, 868–882.

[97] Valikangas, L., Pekkala, E., Larmas, M., Risteli, J., Salo, T., & Tjaderhane, L. (2001). The effects of high levels of glucose and insulin on type I collagen synthesis in mature human odontoblasts and pulp tissue in vitro. *Advances in Dental Research*, 15, 72–75.

[98] Silva-Sousa, Y. T., Peres, L. C., & Foss, M. C. (2003). Are there structural alterations in the enamel organ of offspring of rats with alloxan-induced diabetes mellitus? *Brazilian Dental Journal*, 14(3), 162–167.

[99] Siudikiene, J., Machiulskiene, V., Nyvad, B., Tenovuo, J., & Nedzelskiene, I. (2008). Dental caries increments and related factors in children with type 1 diabetes mellitus. *Caries Research*, 42(5), 354–362.

Chapter 5

Diabetic Ketoacidosis in the Pediatric Population with Type 1 Diabetes

Michal Cohen, Smadar Shilo, Nehama Zuckerman-Levin and Naim Shehadeh

Additional information is available at the end of the chapter

http://dx.doi.org/10.5772/60592

Abstract

Diabetic ketoacidosis (DKA) is a leading cause of morbidity and mortality in patients with type 1 diabetes (T1DM). Individuals familiar with this complication of diabetes should be able to identify the earliest signs and symptoms and act promptly to prevent further deterioration. However, even in patients with established diabetes, the rates of DKA are considerable. This chapter discusses in detail the various aspects of DKA in the pediatric population with T1DM. The prevalence and regional effects on the prevalence of DKA as well as the specific risk factors, whether disease, patient, or physician related, are reviewed. Patients with DKA experience a condition of starvation despite the abundance of metabolic substrate (i.e., glucose); the pathophysiological mechanisms responsible for the development of DKA are outlined. Next, a detailed discussion of the clinical aspects of DKA is provided. This includes the clinical findings at presentation, the approach to treatment, and potential complications. Prevention is the best method for reducing rates of DKA. Somewhat different factors apply in patients with new-onset diabetes when compared with those with established diabetes and these are reviewed.

Keywords: Diabetic ketoacidosis, pediatrics, type 1 diabetes, epidemiology, treatment

1. Introduction

Diabetic ketoacidosis (DKA) is an acute life-threatening complication of type 1 diabetes (T1DM). Despite our detailed knowledge of this condition, rates of occurrence both in new-onset diabetes and in established diabetes are significant. This chapter will discuss various aspects of DKA in the pediatric population with T1DM, ranging from epidemiology and pathophysiology through the spectrum of clinical considerations, including the clinical presentation, diagnosis, treatment, and complications, and will end with a discussion of the importance and means for prevention of DKA.

Chapter outline:

- Epidemiology of DKA in the pediatric population
- Pathophysiology of DKA
- Clinical presentation and diagnosis of DKA
- DKA Treatment in children
- Complications of pediatric DKA
- Prevention of pediatric DKA
- Conclusion

2. Epidemiology of DKA in the pediatric population

Despite our thorough understanding of the pathophysiology of this potentially life-threatening complication of T1DM, DKA remains a relatively common occurrence in childhood diabetes.

2.1. DKA at diagnosis of T1DM

2.1.1. DKA prevalence

The prevalence of DKA at T1DM diagnosis varies greatly worldwide and ranges between 13% and 80% in different countries [1-11]. A large systematic review of 65 studies including over 29,000 children worldwide found that the lowest prevalences were reported in Sweden, Canada, the Slovak Republic, and Finland and the highest prevalences in the United Arab Emirates, Saudi Arabia, and Romania [1]. Latitude and the regional background incidence of T1DM were negatively associated with the prevalence of DKA [1, 10, 12]. Increased incidence of T1DM has previously been associated with more northern latitudes, although it is unclear whether this represents a true environmental effect or rather reflects ethnic and racial variations between populations [13, 14]. Taken together, these associations suggest that decreased awareness to T1DM and related complications may be a risk factor for DKA at diabetes diagnosis. To further support this, lack of a family history of diabetes was shown to increase the risk of presenting with DKA at diabetes diagnosis [7, 15]. However, despite the increasing incidence of T1DM around the world in recent decades [16], and therefore potentially increased awareness, the prevalence of DKA at diagnosis appears to remain stable [5, 6, 9, 17]. Data from the Search for Diabetes in Youth study (SEARCH), a multicenter US study, found that rates remained stable during 8 years of follow-up for the whole pediatric group as well as when assessing separately the younger children (<4 years of age) and the older children and [9]. They also did not detect any significant gender or ethnicity-specific changes over time.

http://dx.doi.org/10.5772/60592

2.1.2. Risk factors for DKA

The majority of data points to similar rates of DKA at diabetes diagnosis in boys and girls worldwide [7, 9, 11, 12, 15] (Table 1). However, one study based in Germany did suggest a slightly increased prevalence in girls [4] and another suggested increased prevalence in girls when assessing the very young age-group, under 2 years of age [3]. A younger age at diabetes diagnosis is consistently identified as an important risk factor related to DKA at presentation [2, 3, 6, 7, 9, 15, 18]. In a systematic review of 46 studies involving 24,000 children worldwide, younger age was found to be the most common factor associated with increased risk for DKA at diabetes diagnosis [12]. Different age cutoffs between 2 and 5 years of age were used in studies to describe this association. Odds ratios higher than 4 were found for Finnish children under 2 years of age when compared to those 2 years or older [19, 20]. In the SEARCH study increased prevalence of DKA at presentation was detected in children less than 4 years of age, particularly when compared to youth 15–19 years of age [7]. The causes for this increased prevalence in younger children are likely multiple. Younger children are more prone to misdiagnosis when initially presenting with T1DM [21]. This can reflect a lower index of suspicion on the physician's side combined with the difficulty of identifying the classic symptoms in a toddler; infants and young children might not be able to describe symptoms, and findings may be similar to those of other acute illnesses. However, toddlers may actually suffer a more aggressive progression of metabolic decompensation. There is evidence that younger children have a shorter prodromal period [22] as well as a more rapid decline in beta cell reserve after diabetes diagnosis [19, 23]. A lower BMI or weight loss have also been associated with increased risk for DKA at diagnosis in a number of small studies [15, 24]. Children from ethnic minorities are at increased risk for DKA at T1DM onset [12]. In the United States, higher rates of DKA at diagnosis have been recorded in Hispanic and African American youth when compared with non-Hispanic white North-American youth [9]. In the UK, children from an Asian background were at increased risk of presenting with DKA, particularly if under 5 years of age[11]. Another study from the UK demonstrated that children from non-white ethnicity were at higher risk of a delayed T1DM diagnosis and that a delayed diagnosis was associated with increased risk of DKA at presentation [25]. In the Israeli Negev, the prevalence of DKA at diabetes diagnosis was significantly higher in the Bedouin minority when compared to either the general population or the Jewish population [26]. In another study from Israel, children from an Ethiopian origin had an increased prevalence of DKA at presentation [15]. However, this is not supported by all studies, and others did not find a predilection to minority groups [7, 27]. Another predictor of DKA is a lower socioeconomic status [28]. Several components of the socioeconomic status have been identified as significant. Lower household income was found in US and Canadian studies to be a risk factor [2, 7, 9]; however, European studies did not necessarily support this [29]. In the United States, lack of private health insurance was also identified [7, 9, 30]. More years of parental education as well as academic education of the parents were found protective [7, 31, 32]. However, even in the more privileged populations, the rate of DKA at diagnosis of diabetes is substantial and recorded to occur in over 20% of patients [7]. "Physician-dependent" factors may also increase the risk for DKA at diabetes diagnosis. Such factors include delayed diagnosis of diabetes or a missed diagnosis [25, 21], delayed presentation to secondary care, or delayed treatment after T1DM diagnosis [10, 17].

Risk factors for diabetic ketoacidosis at diabetes diagnosis	
Patient specific	Younger age
	Ethnic minority
	Lower socioeconomic status
Physician related	Delayed diabetes diagnosis
	Delayed initiation of treatment
Epidemiological	Lower regional background prevalence of T1DM
	Residence in a less northern latitude
Risk factors for recurrent diabetic ketoacidosis	
	Insulin omission and poor adherence to treatment
	Poor metabolic control
	Previous episodes of DKA
	Behavioral and psychiatric disorders
	Higher levels of family conflict
	Lower socioeconomic status
	Limited access to outpatient diabetes care

Table 1. Risk factors for diabetic ketoacidosis in the pediatric population

2.2. DKA in patients with established T1DM

Recurrent DKA is by large a preventable complication in patients with established T1DM. In a large cohort of 1243 children with T1DM, the incidence of DKA in patients with established T1DM was 8/100 person-years [33]. Another study assessing a large database of children with established T1DM from Germany and Austria evaluated the incidence of DKA in the most recent year of follow-up [34]. They found that 6% of children suffered from DKA, 5% had a single episode, and 1% had two or more episodes. Two smaller studies followed children with T1DM for about 8 years and found 20–28% to experience at least one episode of DKA [26, 35]. As reflected in these data, it is estimated that it is the same small proportion of patients (around 20%) that account for the majority of admissions for DKA [33, 36]. Insulin omission and poor adherence to treatment are major risk factors [37] (Table 1). Poorer diabetes control, higher hemoglobin A1c, higher insulin doses, and previous episodes of DKA are also important risk factors [33, 34, 38]. Recurrent DKA episodes peak in teenage years, particularly in females [33, 34]. Moreover, the incidence of DKA was found to increase with age in females, yet remained stable in males. A study evaluating the role of patient and family psychosocial functioning as predictors of recurrent acute diabetic complications [35] found girls with recurrent DKA to demonstrate lower social competence and higher rates of behavioral problems. The families exhibited higher levels of family conflict and decreased family cohesion and organization. Major psychiatric disorders have also been implicated in recurrent DKA [39]. As is the case in DKA at T1DM diagnosis, lower socioeconomic status and limited access to outpatient diabetes care are also predictors of recurrent DKA [39].

http://dx.doi.org/10.5772/60592

3. Pathophysiology of DKA in children

By definition, hyperglycemia and ketoacidosis are the major components of DKA [40]. The initial impairment leading to DKA is an absolute or relative insulin deficiency. The sequence of events that follows leads to a patient that suffers hyperglycemia, dehydration, acidosis, electrolyte deficiencies, and variable degrees of cerebral dysfunction [41] (Figure 1). In a patient with new-onset diabetes, the cause for the insulin deficiency is the progressive deterioration in beta cell reserve and function [42]. In patients with established diabetes, insulin omission (intentional, as a result of insulin pump failure or other technical problems, or related to lack of access to medical care) is a major cause. Acute stress, commonly induced by an intercurrent illness, might precipitate DKA. During stress, counterregulatory hormone (glucagon, cortisol, growth hormone, and epinephrine) levels increase, causing hyperglycemia and an increased requirement for insulin. If this increased need for insulin is not met, DKA may ensue. Furthermore, an acute illness may impair the child's ability to replace fluid losses.

Insulin deficiency leads to hyperglycemia as a result of decreased utilization of glucose at the same time of increased hepatic and renal glucose production. Hyperglycemia increases serum osmolality, and in response, thirst is induced and osmotic diuresis occurs. The increased fluid loss further promotes polydipsia. Because of the unavailability of glucose to tissues, compensatory mechanisms are activated. Counterregulatory hormones are secreted, leading to increased glucose production by gluconeogenesis and glycogenolysis [43]. Insulin resistance increases and lipolysis is promoted, resulting in production of free fatty acids (FFAs). FFAs are metabolized into ketone bodies, particularly β-hydroxybutyrate, by the liver as an alternative energy source. The accumulation of ketones leads to metabolic acidosis. Another result of the decreased insulin and elevated counterregulatory hormone levels is proteolysis and reduced production of proteins. By this mechanism, substrates for gluconeogenesis are added, further contributing to the hyperglycemia. Initially, plasma ketone body levels rise, causing ketonemia and a base deficit; compensating mechanisms are activated and might lead to measurement of a normal pH. As the condition progresses, ketones further accumulate, ketonuria occurs, and eventually the metabolic acidosis becomes evident. The ketoacidosis causes decreased bowel motility, particularly of the small bowl, accompanied by nausea and vomiting. At this stage, the patient may be unable to compensate for the urinary fluid losses. In a vicious cycle, dehydration impairs the renal ability to clear glucose and ketoacids, thus further worsening the hyperglycemia and acidosis. The increasing osmolality, dehydration, and acidosis decrease cerebral function. This might be manifested as lethargy, or even an altered level of consciousness, further impairing the patient's ability to rehydrate. At presentation, the degree of dehydration ranges from mild to severe, with the majority of children presenting with moderate degrees of dehydration [44]. To compensate for the acidosis, respiratory mechanisms are activated, causing the labored, rapid, deep breathing typically described in patients with DKA (i.e., Kussmaul respirations). The acetone released in the breath results in a characteristic fruity odor.

Serum hyperglycemia and hyperosmolarity together with the acidosis and osmotic diuresis lead to significant electrolyte deficiencies and imbalances [40, 45, 46].

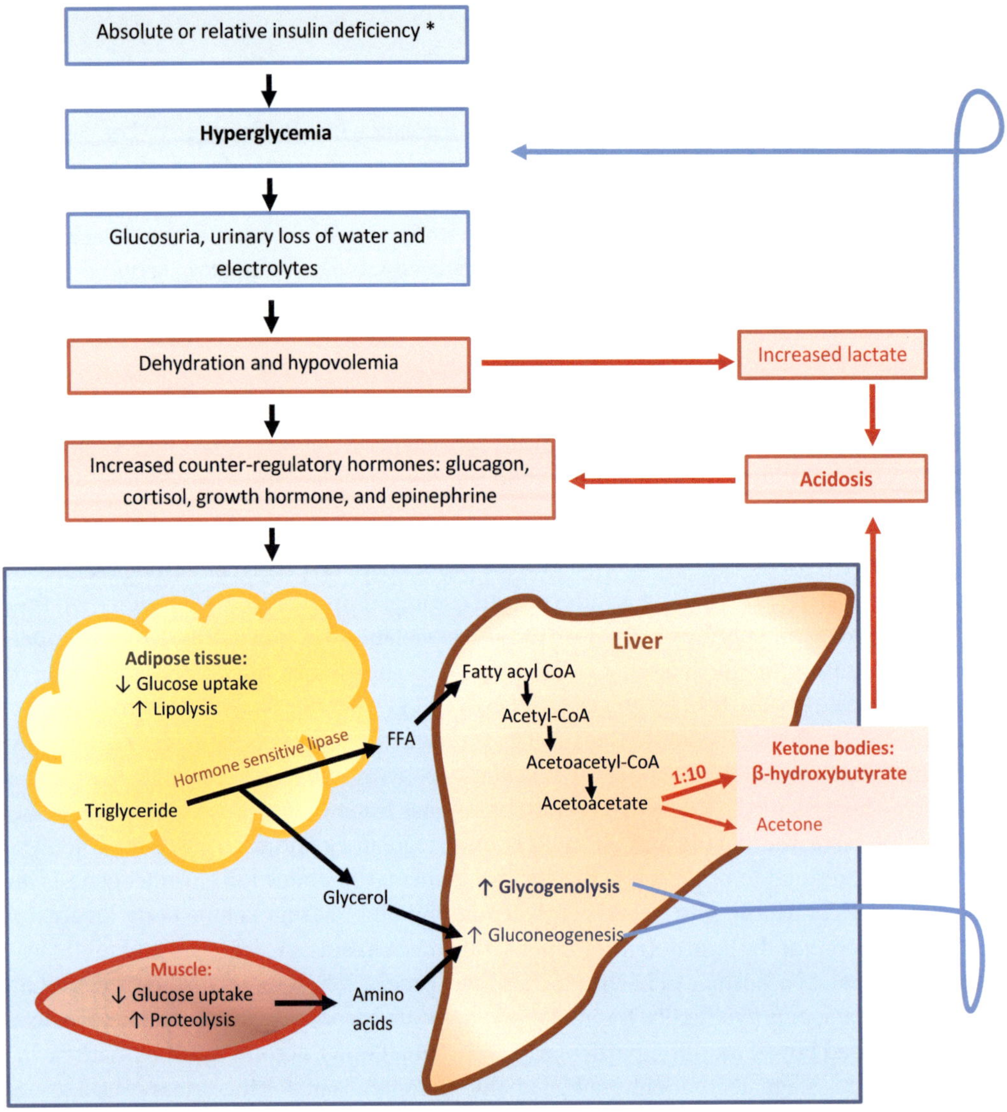

* May be induced by stress, infection, or inadequate insulin dosing in a patient with diabetes. FFA = free fatty acids.

Figure 1. Pathophysiology of diabetic ketoacidosis.

3.1. Potassium depletion

Total body stores of potassium are depleted in basically every patient with DKA, and the average potassium loss is 5 mmol/kg body weight. However, the serum potassium levels may not reflect these losses, and the actual level may be low, normal, or even elevated, particularly if renal function is impaired. The entry of hydrogen ions, accumulated extracellularly due to the acidosis, into cells drives out the intracellular potassium. The osmotic diuresis together with the high levels of aldosterone secreted as a result of the dehydration cause significant

http://dx.doi.org/10.5772/60592

urinary loss of potassium. Emesis might cause further loss of potassium through the gastrointestinal tract. However, an exception is patients with severe volume depletion, in whom renal insufficiency may lead to hyperkalemia. During treatment of DKA, both the insulin itself and the reversal of acidosis generate a net shift of potassium back into cells. Moreover, there is some evidence suggesting a kaliuretic effect of insulin [47]. Altogether, these may result in severe hypokalemia. Patients with hypokalemia at presentation likely suffer more severe total body potassium depletion and are at particular risk of severe hypokalemia and cardiac instability as treatment is provided.

3.2. Sodium and chloride depletion

The osmotic diuresis in DKA results in urinary loss of sodium, and the hyperosmolar state drives water out of cells into the extracellular space, leading to dilutional hyponatremia. The average sodium loss is 6 mmol/kg body weight. Chloride is secreted in the urine with sodium, and the loss is on average 4 mmol/kg body weight. It should be kept in mind that the administration of chloride during the treatment of DKA may lead to hyperchloremic metabolic acidosis, thus interfering with the correction of acidosis.

3.3. Phosphate depletion

Phosphate shifted extracellularly by the acidosis is then lost in the urine. Phosphate losses can be substantial and are estimated to be about 0.5–2.5 mmol/kg body weight. Significant hypophosphatemia has the potential to impair oxygen delivery to tissues and cause muscle weakness. However, despite very low serum levels of phosphate in some patients, such complications are rare, and studies did not demonstrate a benefit for phosphorous replacement [48, 49].

Beyond the electrolyte deficiencies described, in recent years, several studies have pointed out that a deficiency of thiamine (vitamin B1), a water-soluble vitamin of the B complex, may be clinically significant in patients with DKA. Thiamine deficiency was found to be common in children with DKA and may worsen with treatment [50]. The role of this deficiency in the clinical presentation of DKA is yet to be revealed.

4. Clinical presentation and diagnosis of DKA

Metabolic decompensation in DKA usually develops over a period of hours to a few days. Progression can be particularly rapid in patients with established diabetes. Misdiagnosis of a patient with new-onset diabetes may lead to deterioration of the metabolic status. Particularly in young children, misdiagnosis may be a result of the nonspecific symptoms and signs often described in DKA. The earliest clinical manifestations of DKA are related to hyperglycemia and may differ according to age, length of prodromal period, degree of acidosis, and volume depletion [51, 52]. Symptoms and signs in DKA are most often related to the hyperglycemia, dehydration, and acidosis [4, 53-55].

4.1. Symptoms

- Polydipsia, polyuria, and/or nocturia are almost always present, although often not reported.
- Nocturnal or daytime secondary enuresis is often described; polyphagia and weight loss may occur.
- As a result of the acidosis, patients may suffer nausea, vomiting, abdominal pain, shortness of breath, lethargy, or fatigue.

4.2. Physical signs

- Dehydration: Children with DKA often present with 5–10% fluid deficit [51, 56]. They may lack the classical signs of hypovolemia and dehydration because of the acute and chronic losses of both extracellular and intracellular water [57]. Findings depend on the degree of dehydration and may include dry oral mucosa and decreased skin turgor, tachycardia, a sunken fontanelle, and/or sunken eyes. Most patients are normotensive, although postural hypotension can occur.
- Tachypnea or Kussmaul (deep, sighing, and labored) respiration with a fruity acetone odor.
- Signs of decreased tissue perfusion such as a slow capillary refill.
- Neurologic findings [58]: from confusion and drowsiness to decreased consciousness and coma. Neurologic findings should raise the suspicion of cerebral edema.

In infants, especially those who are not toilet trained, the diagnosis may be delayed. Weight loss, irritability, and decreased activity are common at presentation. Dehydration and severe diaper rash may be the only physical signs. Older children and adolescents can manifest profound wasting, cachexia, and prostration on DKA presentation, especially with a prolonged course of uncontrolled/misdiagnosed diabetes.

4.3. Laboratory findings

4.3.1. Diagnostic criteria

Biochemical criteria for the diagnosis of DKA are defined as follows [40, 51, 56, 59]:

- Hyperglycemia: blood glucose (BG) >200 mg/dl (11 mmol/L)
- Metabolic acidosis: venous pH <7.3 and/or bicarbonate <15 mmol/L
- Ketonemia and ketonuria: serum beta hydroxybutyrate ≥3 mmol/L

On certain occasions, patients may present with "euglycemic ketoacidosis" where glucose levels are near normal [54, 59]. This may develop in young children who consumed small amounts of carbohydrates or are partially treated or in children with emesis.

The severity of DKA is established by the degree of acidosis: mild DKA, pH 7.2–7.3 or bicarbonate <15 mmol/L; moderate DKA, pH 7.1–7.2 or bicarbonate 5–10 mmol/L; and severe

DKA, pH <7.1 or bicarbonate <5 mmol/L [51, 56, 58]. The duration of symptoms, volume deficit, degree of ketosis, and neurologic status further determine the severity of illness in a child with DKA.

4.3.2. Acid–base balance

Acidosis is caused by the production and accumulation of ketones in the serum [49]. Three ketones are produced in DKA: two ketoacids (beta-hydroxybutyrate and acetoacetate) and the neutral ketone, acetone. In DKA, beta-hydroxybutyrate constitutes 75% of the circulating ketones. During recovery, it is converted to acetoacetate and acetone, which persists for a longer period. Therefore, measuring serum beta-hydroxybutyrate is the most useful for diagnosis. The severity of the metabolic acidosis is dependent on the compensatory respiratory alkalosis, the acid excretion in the urine [60], and the duration and rate of increased ketoacid production. The serum anion gap (AG) is an index of unmeasured anions in the blood (normal in children is 12 ± 2 mEq/L). Most patients with DKA present with a high AG (≥20 mEq/L) due to high serum levels of ketoacids. The resolution of ketoacidosis is followed by a normal AG.

4.3.3. Electrolyte imbalances

Laboratory tests that should be routinely monitored in the setting of DKA include serum glucose, electrolytes, creatinine and BUN, blood gases, pH, bicarbonate, and a complete blood count. Changes over time in electrolytes and renal function tests must be followed.

Serum potassium: As mentioned earlier, potassium loss can be a result of increased ketoacid excretion, osmotic diuresis, vomiting, or diarrhea. The serum potassium concentration may be normal, increased, or decreased at diagnosis of DKA. However, monitoring of potassium levels is crucial because hypokalemia may eventually develop.

Serum sodium: Low serum sodium in DKA may occur due to hyperglycemia and its effect on plasma osmolarity. Polydipsia and excessive consumption of water can also contribute to lowering sodium concentration. Osmotic dieresis and water loss in excess of sodium and potassium will tend to raise the serum sodium concentration. Hyperlipidemia can cause pseudohyponatremia [61].

Serum phosphate: Decreased phosphate intake and phosphaturia may result in a negative phosphate balance. At presentation of DKA, serum phosphate is usually normal or high due to the combined effect of metabolic acidosis and insulin deficiency. The degree of phosphate loss in DKA is apparent after insulin treatment [62].

4.4. Differential diagnosis of DKA

DKA should be differentiated from other causes of acidosis and/or hyperglycemia, such as acute gastroenteritis with metabolic acidosis, uremia, salicylate intoxication, starvation ketosis and lactic acidosis. When the presenting symptom is altered consciousness or coma, encephalitis and other CNS pathologies must be ruled out. Diabetic ketoacidosis should also be distinguished from the hyperosmolar hyperglycemic state, which is infrequent in children [51, 57, 63]. The main differences between these conditions are the degree of acidosis and insulinopenia.

5. DKA treatment in children

Successful treatment of DKA requires correction of dehydration, acid–base and electrolyte imbalances, insulin administration, and identification of comorbid and precipitating conditions. This treatment may be associated with inherent risks of inducing hypoglycemia, hypokalemia, and cerebral edema. Therefore, any protocol must be used with caution, and close monitoring of patients is crucial. Children with severe DKA, an altered level of consciousness, or those who are at increased risk for complications should be considered for treatment in an intensive care setting. In this chapter, we will focus on the general principals and considerations in DKA management as well as controversies regarding DKA treatment.

5.1. Standard protocols for DKA management

There is some variability in protocols for DKA management, but the basic principles are similar in the various protocols available in the literature [40, 51, 64, 65]. Protocols enabling standardization of treatment are of great value to the treating team involved; however, clinical judgment should always be practiced. Frequent monitoring of the patient is a very important aspect of the treatment and should include meticulous documentation of clinical observations, fluid balance, laboratory results, and medications administered. A neurological follow-up for warning signs and symptoms of cerebral edema is also essential.

5.2. Fluid replacement

Fluid replacement in children with DKA remains a controversial topic with regard to the amount of intravenous fluid, rate of delivery, and fluid composition. Current recommendations are based on expert consensus statements and accumulated clinical experience, as evidence from large randomized clinical trials is lacking.

5.2.1. First hour fluid resuscitation

The goals of initial volume expansion are to restore the effective circulating volume and the glomerular filtration rate. Intravenous fluid administration bares the risk of inducing an elevation in the intracranial pressure (ICP), potentially resulting in cerebral edema, and thus should be done carefully [66, 67]. In a rabbit model of DKA, the use of hypotonic fluids, compared with isotonic, was associated with greater rises in ICP [66]. Some studies suggest that rapid fluid replacement may increase the risk of cerebral edema [68, 69], although other studies did not support this finding [70, 71]. Studies in both adults and children demonstrated a more rapid correction of acidosis when a slower rate of fluid administration with isotonic or near-isotonic solutions was used [72, 73]. Hyperchloremic metabolic acidosis is another often overlooked risk resulting from the use of large volumes of normal saline (NS) (0.9%) [73, 74]. At present, there is no data that support the use of colloid in preference to crystalloid in the treatment of DKA. Based on these data, most protocols recommend an initial IV infusion of 10–20 ml/kg of normal saline (NS) (0.9%) or Ringer's lactate over the first 1 to 2 h of treatment. Fluid boluses may be repeated according to the patient's hemodynamic status. However, total IV fluids should not exceed 40 ml/kg in the initial 4 h of treatment due to the aforementioned risks.

5.2.2. Fluid replacement over the next 24–48 h of treatment

Once the child is hemodynamically stable, subsequent volume expansion should be given more gradually, with a goal of replacing the remaining fluid deficit over the next 24 to 72 h. Significant additional fluid loss after initiation of treatment is rare because vomiting and excessive urine output usually resolve within the first hours of treatment. Half NS or NS (0.45–0.9%) solutions are appropriate for replacement. The rate of fluid administration is guided by the estimated degree of dehydration and fluid deficit. Calculating the effective osmolality is also of use, and most often, replacement is in the range of 1.5–2 times the usual maintenance requirement based on age and weight. Unless a contraindication exists, potassium must be added at this time (see below). To prevent a rapid decrease in plasma glucose concentration and hypoglycemia, 5% glucose should be added to the IV fluid when the plasma glucose falls to approximately 250–300 mg/dl (14–17 mmol/L), or sooner if rapidly decreasing. Fluids that were given in another facility before assessment should be factored into calculation of deficit and be subtracted from the 24-h totals.

5.3. Insulin administration

5.3.1. Intravenous insulin administration

Insulin therapy is essential to suppress lipolysis and ketogenesis and to correct acidosis. Insulin infusion is recommended 1–2 h after starting fluid replacement therapy and initial volume expansion. An initial IV bolus of insulin is unnecessary, it was not shown to affect the duration of time to attaining a serum glucose level of less than 250 mg/dl, yet it may increase the risk of cerebral edema [69, 75, 76]. A slow infusion of a low dose of 0.1 U/kg/h IV insulin is considered the standard of care in pediatric DKA [77, 78]. The dose of insulin should remain 0.1 U/kg/h at least until the resolution of DKA (pH >7.30; bicarbonate >15 mmol/L and/or closure of the anion gap). It is possible that even a lower dose of insulin is sufficient for DKA treatment. A recent randomized control trial compared a very low dose IV insulin infusion (0.05 U/kg/hr) to the standard dose. Similar results were achieved in terms of the rate of blood glucose decrease and the resolution of acidosis, suggesting that a dose lower than the current standard dose can be used [78].

5.3.2. Subcutaneous insulin regimens

Few studies, mostly in adults, demonstrated subcutaneous rapid acting insulin injected every 1–2 h to be a valid alternative for the standard intravenous insulin treatment of mild-to-moderate uncomplicated DKA [79, 80]. In our practice, we administer subcutaneous regular insulin (SCRI) every 4 h for treating children with DKA and pH ≥7.00 and K >2.5 mEq/L. Insulin therapy is initiated during the second hour of treatment and administered every 4 h until resolution of DKA. The insulin dose is calculated as 0.8–1 IU/kg/day divided by 6. This treatment was found to be a simple, effective, and safe alternative to the standard DKA protocol. Such treatment has the potential to simplify insulin administration and reduce both patient inconvenience and admission costs. Subcutaneous insulin should not be used in subjects whose peripheral circulation is impaired.

5.4. Electrolyte replacements

5.4.1. Potassium replacement

Children with DKA suffer from total body potassium deficits of approximately 3–6 mmol/kg. Hypokalemia at presentation may be related to prolonged duration of disease, whereas hyperkalemia primarily results from reduced renal function [60]. Insulin administration and the correction of acidosis drive potassium back into the cells, which may cause hypokalemia and predispose the patient to cardiac arrhythmias. Replacement therapy is usually required regardless of the serum potassium concentration. In most protocols, potassium is not given during the first hour of fluid resuscitation unless the patient is hypokalemic, in which case some protocols recommend adding potassium to the initial volume expansion before starting insulin therapy. Potassium can be given as potassium phosphate or potassium chloride. The starting potassium concentration in the infusate should be 40 mmol/L. Subsequent potassium therapy should be based on serum potassium measurements.

5.4.2. Phosphate and calcium replacement

Prospective studies have not shown clinical benefit from phosphate replacement [48, 49, 81]. The deficit usually corrects spontaneously, although it should be kept in mind that it may persist for several days after the resolution of DKA [45]. Therefore, only severe and symptomatic hypophosphatemia accompanied by significant weakness should be treated with phosphate supplements. Potassium phosphate may be used safely in combination with potassium chloride or acetate to avoid hyperchloremia. Careful monitoring of serum calcium should be performed to avoid hypocalcemia. In a study on nine children with DKA, during phosphate infusion, transient hypocalcemia occurred in 67% and transient hypomagnesemia in 56%. One child developed carpopedal spasms refractory to intravenous infusion of calcium gluconate but responsive to intramuscular injection of magnesium sulfate. In 33%, parathyroid hormone was low at the time of hypocalcemia, an observation that suggests transient hypoparathyroidism [82].

5.4.3. Bicarbonate therapy

Acidosis is reversible by insulin replacement. Several clinical trials have shown no clinical benefit from bicarbonate administration in pediatric DKA [83-86]. Moreover, bicarbonate therapy may cause paradoxical CNS acidosis. Bicarbonate crosses the blood–brain barrier slowly, yet the CO_2 formed ($HCO_3 + H+ \rightarrow H_2O + CO_2$) crosses rapidly into the CNS forming

H_2CO_3, thus worsening the CNS acidosis [87, 88]. As a result of the sodium supplement included in the bicarbonate preparations, this therapy may be associated with hypokalemia and increasing osmolality. Bicarbonate administration was also reported as a risk factor for cerebral edema in several studies [51, 69, 89]. Despite all the risks mentioned, in must be kept in mind that patients with severe acidemia (arterial pH ≤6.9) in whom decreased cardiac contractility and peripheral vasodilatation can further impair tissue perfusion and patients with life-threatening hyperkalemia may benefit from cautious alkali therapy [84]. If bicarbonate is considered necessary, it should be cautiously administered at a dose of 1–2 mmol/kg over 60 min.

5.5. Introduction of oral fluids and transition to SC insulin injections

Upon resolution of DKA and when substantial clinical improvement has occurred, oral fluids can be introduced and a protocol of subcutaneous insulin can be initiated or restarted.

6. Complications of pediatric DKA

As mentioned in detail earlier, diabetic ketoacidosis (DKA) is treated with fluids, electrolytes, and insulin. With prompt treatment, complications of DKA are uncommon. However, when complications do occur, they are usually serious with significant mortality and long-term morbidity. Surprisingly, the most common complication of DKA (cerebral edema) may be related to this lifesaving treatment.

6.1. Cerebral edema

Cerebral edema is a devastating and unpredictable complication of DKA and its treatment. Epidemiological studies demonstrate that overall cerebral edema occurs in around 7/1000 episodes of DKA and is more common in children and newly diagnosed patients. Other studies found that clinically apparent cerebral edema develops in 1–2% of children with DKA [90]. The pathophysiology of cerebral edema is not well understood, and it is likely that several processes contribute to the development of this complication: ischemic, osmotic, and vasogenic.

Osmotic: ultimately, cerebral edema is due to excessive entry of water into the cells of the central nervous system due to the presence of intracellular idiogenic osmoles causing swelling of the brain as serum osmolality drops during treatment.

Vasogenic: studies using magnetic resonance diffusion weighted imaging demonstrate that the apparent diffusion coefficient of brain water is greater during treatment of DKA than during recovery, indicating increased extracellular fluid due to an increase in blood brain barrier permeability during the acute treatment phase of DKA [91-93]. These findings are consistent with the vasogenic cerebral edema, i.e., fluid surrounding the cells, rather than osmotic cell swelling that has previously been suggested. This vasogenic theory is also supported by the fact that the degrees of dehydration and hyperventilation at presentation, but not initial osmolality or osmotic changes during treatment, were correlated with degree of edema formation [92]. This edema (within the enclosed space of the cranium) can cause transtentorial brain herniation through the foramen magnum, leading to unconsciousness and respiratory arrest.

6.1.1. Risk factors for cerebral edema

Several case–control studies have pointed out risk factors for the development of cerebral edema [69, 70, 94, 95]. These can be divided into two main groups.

Risk factors related to disease severity at presentation:

a. Younger age

b. Newly diagnosed compared with established diabetes

c. More severe acidosis at presentation

d. Higher serum urea levels

e. Lower partial arterial CO_2 ($PaCO_2$) values

Risk factors related to therapy:

a. Larger volume of fluid given during the first 4 h of treatment

b. Administration of bicarbonate

c. Lower plasma sodium concentrations

d. Administration of insulin within the first hour of treatment

6.1.2. Symptoms and signs

These typically appear within 6–24 h after starting intravenous fluids and insulin treatment. Therefore, it is crucial to monitor and recognize the early warning signs of cerebral edema through careful monitoring of all DKA patients. These include signs and symptoms of increasing intracranial pressure, such as a decline in the level of consciousness, headaches, bradycardia, depressed respiration and apnea, papillary changes, papilledema, posturing, seizures, and coma.

6.1.3. Diagnosis

The diagnosis of cerebral edema is clinical. Recognition of the above-mentioned signs and symptoms should allow early intervention and hopefully prevention of morbidities associated with this condition. CT or MRI of the brain should be performed to rule out other diagnoses and potentially confirm the diagnosis of cerebral edema. However, it should be emphasized that radiographic imaging may be unhelpful in detecting cerebral edema if performed very early after the development of symptoms.

6.1.4. Treatment of cerebral edema

The patient should be treated and monitored in the intensive care unit; however, if located elsewhere, initial treatment must not be delayed until transitioned. Mannitol or hypertonic saline should be readily available for use at the earliest signs and symptoms of cerebral edema. Other measures include a reduction in the rate of fluid administration and elevation of the head of the bed. Mannitol 1 g/kg (5 ml/kg of mannitol 20%) should be administered over 15 min; alternatively, hypertonic saline (3% NaCl) 5–10 ml/kg over 30 min can be administered. This treatment will reduce brain edema and blood viscosity and improve cerebral blood flow. Intubation and ventilation may be necessary to provide adequate ventilation and correct acidosis. Aggressive hyperventilation has been associated with poor neurological outcome and is not recommended [96].

6.2. Hypoglycemia and hypokalemia

These are additional potential complications of DKA treatment. Both are discussed earlier in the chapter.

6.3. Rare complications of DKA

6.3.1. Adult respiratory distress syndrome

This has been reported in patients with DKA, especially in patients younger than 50 years. Clinical features include dyspnea and tachypnea, with central cyanosis and nonspecific chest symptoms.

6.3.2. Acute renal failure

This can develop due to severe dehydration. Once fluid replacement is restored, kidney function should start to recover.

6.3.3. Thromboembolic complications

These may arise as a consequence of dehydration, increased blood viscosity, and coagulability. Rehydration and restoration of body fluids might help in preventing these complications [97]. Established thromboembolic complication should be treated promptly.

7. Prevention of pediatric DKA

The best approach for decreasing the burden of DKA is prevention. Preventive measures are based on the identified risk factors of T1DM and DKA and on their clinical presentation. Risk factors differ between DKA at the time of T1DM diagnosis and episodes occurring in patients with established diabetes. Identifying high-risk children, using both immunologic and genetic methods, can lead to earlier diagnosis of diabetes and decreased DKA incidence at disease onset [10, 33, 98, 99]. However, such screening raises obvious ethical questions, as the exact risk or timing of the development of diabetes in a child at risk are not known and no treatment has proved protective thus far. In families with T1DM, a special attention to early symptoms and signs is recommended to detect the onset of diabetes in other members and to prevent future DKA [51].

Greater public awareness to signs and symptoms of DKA has been related to decreased rates of DKA. This is further emphasized by the success of awareness campaigns in decreasing the rates of DKA. A campaign to increase awareness of physicians, schools, and parents was carried out in Parma, Italy [1991–1997] [100, 101]. The researchers displayed posters in pediatric centers, schools, and physician offices and demonstrated a significant reduction in the DKA rate from 78% to 12% in 6–14 years old children over an 8-year period. An Australian study demonstrated a reduction in DKA prevalence in new-onset diabetes from 38% to 14%, when repeating the Parma study diabetes awareness campaign [102]. However, it is important to mention that not all such programs have been successful [5], and complex risk factors might be involved.

The rates of DKA in patients with established diabetes can also be reduced. Identifying the specific causes for recurrent DKA in a child is important and may prevent future DKA events [40]. Detailed and intensive diabetes education programs, telephone help lines, and availability of skilled health care providers can reduce DKA occurrence [103-106]. Education programs lead to better understanding of the disease and might assist families in identifying times of increased risk (i.e., intercurrent illness or pump malfunction) as well as early signs of deterioration and of DKA. Such programs are important to the noncompliant children, especially those with recurrent episodes of DKA, and should be led by professional teams [17, 107]. Education and adult guidance were shown to decrease insulin omission in patients with recurrent DKA episodes [108]. Early identification of ketosis, using home measurement of beta-hydroxybutyrate, can prevent progression to DKA [109].

8. Conclusion

DKA is a serious complication of pediatric T1DM. The pathophysiology is complex, demonstrating reciprocal effects between the metabolic derangements involved. A "hunger" response takes place despite the abundance of metabolic substrate. Various risk factors have been identified, some are patient related yet others emphasize the important effects of both family and social circumstances. DKA is largely preventable, and efforts to further increase awareness to this complication of diabetes should be encouraged.

Author details

Michal Cohen[1*], Smadar Shilo[1], Nehama Zuckerman-Levin[1,2] and Naim Shehadeh[1,2]

*Address all correspondence to: cohenm4@gmail.com

1 Pediatric Diabetes Clinic and Pediatrics A Division, the Ruth Rappaport Children's Hospital, Rambam healthcare campus, Haifa, Israel

2 Rappaport Faculty of Medicine, Technion, Haifa, Israel

http://dx.doi.org/10.5772/60592

References

[1] Usher-Smith JA, Thompson M, Ercole A, Walter FM. Variation between countries in the frequency of diabetic ketoacidosis at first presentation of type 1 diabetes in children: a systematic review. Diabetologia. 2012;55(11):2878-94. Epub 2012/08/31.

[2] Bui H, To T, Stein R, Fung K, Daneman D. Is diabetic ketoacidosis at disease onset a result of missed diagnosis? The Journal of pediatrics. 2010;156(3):472-7. Epub 2009/12/08.

[3] Schober E, Rami B, Waldhoer T, Austrian Diabetes Incidence Study G. Diabetic ketoacidosis at diagnosis in Austrian children in 1989-2008: a population-based analysis. Diabetologia. 2010;53(6):1057-61. Epub 2010/03/10.

[4] Neu A, Willasch A, Ehehalt S, Hub R, Ranke MB, Baden-Wuerttemberg DG. Ketoacidosis at onset of type 1 diabetes mellitus in children--frequency and clinical presentation. Pediatric diabetes. 2003;4(2):77-81. Epub 2003/12/06.

[5] Fritsch M, Schober E, Rami-Merhar B, Hofer S, Frohlich-Reiterer E, Waldhoer T, et al. Diabetic ketoacidosis at diagnosis in Austrian children: a population-based analysis, 1989-2011. The Journal of pediatrics. 2013;163(5):1484-8 e1. Epub 2013/08/21.

[6] Lansdown AJ, Barton J, Warner J, Williams D, Gregory JW, Harvey JN, et al. Prevalence of ketoacidosis at diagnosis of childhood onset Type 1 diabetes in Wales from 1991 to 2009 and effect of a publicity campaign. Diabetic medicine : a journal of the British Diabetic Association. 2012;29(12):1506-9. Epub 2012/03/15.

[7] Rewers A, Klingensmith G, Davis C, Petitti DB, Pihoker C, Rodriguez B, et al. Presence of diabetic ketoacidosis at diagnosis of diabetes mellitus in youth: the Search for Diabetes in Youth Study. Pediatrics. 2008;121(5):e1258-66. Epub 2008/05/03.

[8] Kamal Alanani NM, Alsulaimani AA. Epidemiological pattern of newly diagnosed children with type 1 diabetes mellitus, Taif, Saudi Arabia. TheScientificWorldJournal. 2013;2013:421569. Epub 2013/11/14.

[9] Dabelea D, Rewers A, Stafford JM, Standiford DA, Lawrence JM, Saydah S, et al. Trends in the prevalence of ketoacidosis at diabetes diagnosis: the SEARCH for diabetes in youth study. Pediatrics. 2014;133(4):e938-45. Epub 2014/04/02.

[10] Levy-Marchal C, Patterson CC, Green A, Europe EASG, Diabetes. Geographical variation of presentation at diagnosis of type I diabetes in children: the EURODIAB study. European and Dibetes. Diabetologia. 2001;44 Suppl 3:B75-80. Epub 2001/11/29.

[11] Alvi NS, Davies P, Kirk JM, Shaw NJ. Diabetic ketoacidosis in Asian children. Archives of disease in childhood. 2001;85(1):60-1. Epub 2001/06/23.

[12] Usher-Smith JA, Thompson MJ, Sharp SJ, Walter FM. Factors associated with the presence of diabetic ketoacidosis at diagnosis of diabetes in children and young adults: a systematic review. Bmj. 2011;343:d4092. Epub 2011/07/09.

[13] Karvonen M, Tuomilehto J, Libman I, LaPorte R. A review of the recent epidemiological data on the worldwide incidence of type 1 (insulin-dependent) diabetes mellitus.

World Health Organization DIAMOND Project Group. Diabetologia. 1993;36(10): 883-92. Epub 1993/10/01.

[14] Karvonen M, Viik-Kajander M, Moltchanova E, Libman I, LaPorte R, Tuomilehto J. Incidence of childhood type 1 diabetes worldwide. Diabetes Mondiale (DiaMond) Project Group. Diabetes care. 2000;23(10):1516-26. Epub 2000/10/07.

[15] de Vries L, Oren L, Lazar L, Lebenthal Y, Shalitin S, Phillip M. Factors associated with diabetic ketoacidosis at onset of Type 1 diabetes in children and adolescents. Diabetic medicine : a journal of the British Diabetic Association. 2013;30(11):1360-6. Epub 2013/06/14.

[16] Group DP. Incidence and trends of childhood Type 1 diabetes worldwide 1990-1999. Diabetic medicine : a journal of the British Diabetic Association. 2006;23(8):857-66. Epub 2006/08/17.

[17] Lokulo-Sodipe K, Moon RJ, Edge JA, Davies JH. Identifying targets to reduce the incidence of diabetic ketoacidosis at diagnosis of type 1 diabetes in the UK. Archives of disease in childhood. 2014;99(5):438-42. Epub 2014/01/08.

[18] Savoldelli RD, Farhat SC, Manna TD. Alternative management of diabetic ketoacidosis in a Brazilian pediatric emergency department. Diabetology & metabolic syndrome. 2010;2:41. Epub 2010/06/17.

[19] Komulainen J, Kulmala P, Savola K, Lounamaa R, Ilonen J, Reijonen H, et al. Clinical, autoimmune, and genetic characteristics of very young children with type 1 diabetes. Childhood Diabetes in Finland (DiMe) Study Group. Diabetes care. 1999;22(12): 1950-5. Epub 1999/12/10.

[20] Hekkala A, Knip M, Veijola R. Ketoacidosis at diagnosis of type 1 diabetes in children in northern Finland: temporal changes over 20 years. Diabetes care. 2007;30(4): 861-6. Epub 2007/03/30.

[21] Mallare JT, Cordice CC, Ryan BA, Carey DE, Kreitzer PM, Frank GR. Identifying risk factors for the development of diabetic ketoacidosis in new onset type 1 diabetes mellitus. Clinical pediatrics. 2003;42(7):591-7. Epub 2003/10/14.

[22] Neu A, Ehehalt S, Willasch A, Kehrer M, Hub R, Ranke MB. Varying clinical presentations at onset of type 1 diabetes mellitus in children--epidemiological evidence for different subtypes of the disease? Pediatric diabetes. 2001;2(4):147-53. Epub 2004/03/16.

[23] Sochett EB, Daneman D, Clarson C, Ehrlich RM. Factors affecting and patterns of residual insulin secretion during the first year of type 1 (insulin-dependent) diabetes mellitus in children. Diabetologia. 1987;30(7):453-9. Epub 1987/07/01.

[24] Hekkala A, Reunanen A, Koski M, Knip M, Veijola R, Finnish Pediatric Diabetes R. Age-related differences in the frequency of ketoacidosis at diagnosis of type 1 diabetes in children and adolescents. Diabetes care. 2010;33(7):1500-2. Epub 2010/04/24.

[25] Sundaram PC, Day E, Kirk JM. Delayed diagnosis in type 1 diabetes mellitus. Archives of disease in childhood. 2009;94(2):151-2. Epub 2008/06/20.

[26] Hilmi A, Pasternak Y, Friger M, Loewenthal N, Haim A, Hershkovitz E. Ethnic differences in glycemic control and diabetic ketoacidosis rate among children with diabetes mellitus type 1 in the Negev area. The Israel Medical Association journal : IMAJ. 2013;15(6):267-70. Epub 2013/07/26.

[27] Abdul-Rasoul M, Al-Mahdi M, Al-Qattan H, Al-Tarkait N, Alkhouly M, Al-Safi R, et al. Ketoacidosis at presentation of type 1 diabetes in children in Kuwait: frequency and clinical characteristics. Pediatric diabetes. 2010;11(5):351-6. Epub 2009/10/14.

[28] Blanc N, Lucidarme N, Tubiana-Rufi N. [Factors associated with childhood diabetes manifesting as ketoacidosis and its severity]. Archives de pediatrie : organe officiel de la Societe francaise de pediatrie. 2003;10(4):320-5. Epub 2003/06/24. Facteurs associes a l'acidocetose revelatrice du diabete de l'enfant et a sa severite.

[29] Komulainen J, Lounamaa R, Knip M, Kaprio EA, Akerblom HK. Ketoacidosis at the diagnosis of type 1 (insulin dependent) diabetes mellitus is related to poor residual beta cell function. Childhood Diabetes in Finland Study Group. Archives of disease in childhood. 1996;75(5):410-5. Epub 1996/11/01.

[30] Maniatis AK, Goehrig SH, Gao D, Rewers A, Walravens P, Klingensmith GJ. Increased incidence and severity of diabetic ketoacidosis among uninsured children with newly diagnosed type 1 diabetes mellitus. Pediatric diabetes. 2005;6(2):79-83. Epub 2005/06/21.

[31] Rosenbauer J, Icks A, Giani G. Clinical characteristics and predictors of severe ketoacidosis at onset of type 1 diabetes mellitus in children in a North Rhine-Westphalian region, Germany. Journal of pediatric endocrinology & metabolism : JPEM. 2002;15(8):1137-45. Epub 2002/10/22.

[32] Sadauskaite-Kuehne V, Samuelsson U, Jasinskiene E, Padaiga Z, Urbonaite B, Edenvall H, et al. Severity at onset of childhood type 1 diabetes in countries with high and low incidence of the condition. Diabetes research and clinical practice. 2002;55(3): 247-54. Epub 2002/02/19.

[33] Rewers A, Chase HP, Mackenzie T, Walravens P, Roback M, Rewers M, et al. Predictors of acute complications in children with type 1 diabetes. Jama. 2002;287(19): 2511-8. Epub 2002/05/22.

[34] Fritsch M, Rosenbauer J, Schober E, Neu A, Placzek K, Holl RW, et al. Predictors of diabetic ketoacidosis in children and adolescents with type 1 diabetes. Experience from a large multicentre database. Pediatric diabetes. 2011;12(4 Pt 1):307-12. Epub 2011/04/07.

[35] Dumont RH, Jacobson AM, Cole C, Hauser ST, Wolfsdorf JI, Willett JB, et al. Psychosocial predictors of acute complications of diabetes in youth. Diabetic medicine : a journal of the British Diabetic Association. 1995;12(7):612-8. Epub 1995/07/01.

[36] Skinner TC. Recurrent diabetic ketoacidosis: causes, prevention and management. Hormone research. 2002;57 Suppl 1:78-80. Epub 2002/04/30.

[37] Morris AD, Boyle DI, McMahon AD, Greene SA, MacDonald TM, Newton RW. Adherence to insulin treatment, glycaemic control, and ketoacidosis in insulin-dependent diabetes mellitus. The DARTS/MEMO Collaboration. Diabetes Audit and Research in Tayside Scotland. Medicines Monitoring Unit. Lancet. 1997;350(9090):1505-10. Epub 1997/12/06.

[38] Levine BS, Anderson BJ, Butler DA, Antisdel JE, Brackett J, Laffel LM. Predictors of glycemic control and short-term adverse outcomes in youth with type 1 diabetes. The Journal of pediatrics. 2001;139(2):197-203. Epub 2001/08/07.

[39] Rewers M. Challenges in diagnosing type 1 diabetes in different populations. Diabetes & metabolism journal. 2012;36(2):90-7. Epub 2012/04/28.

[40] Wolfsdorf J, Craig ME, Daneman D, Dunger D, Edge J, Lee W, et al. Diabetic ketoacidosis in children and adolescents with diabetes. Pediatric diabetes. 2009;10 Suppl 12:118-33. Epub 2009/09/17.

[41] Foster DW, McGarry JD. The metabolic derangements and treatment of diabetic ketoacidosis. The New England journal of medicine. 1983;309(3):159-69. Epub 1983/07/21.

[42] Matveyenko AV, Butler PC. Relationship between beta-cell mass and diabetes onset. Diabetes, obesity & metabolism. 2008;10 Suppl 4:23-31. Epub 2008/10/18.

[43] Umpierrez GE, DiGirolamo M, Tuvlin JA, Isaacs SD, Bhoola SM, Kokko JP. Differences in metabolic and hormonal milieu in diabetic- and alcohol-induced ketoacidosis. Journal of critical care. 2000;15(2):52-9. Epub 2000/07/06.

[44] Fagan MJ, Avner J, Khine H. Initial fluid resuscitation for patients with diabetic ketoacidosis: how dry are they? Clinical pediatrics. 2008;47(9):851-5. Epub 2008/07/16.

[45] Atchley DW, Loeb RF, Richards DW, Benedict EM, Driscoll ME. ON DIABETIC ACIDOSIS: A Detailed Study of Electrolyte Balances Following the Withdrawal and Reestablishment of Insulin Therapy. The Journal of clinical investigation. 1933;12(2):297-326. Epub 1933/03/01.

[46] Nabarro JD, Spencer AG, Stowers JM. Treatment of diabetic ketosis. Lancet. 1952;1(6716):983-9. Epub 1952/05/17.

[47] Carlotti AP, St George-Hyslop C, Bohn D, Halperin ML. Hypokalemia during treatment of diabetic ketoacidosis: clinical evidence for an aldosterone-like action of insulin. The Journal of pediatrics. 2013;163(1):207-12 e1. Epub 2013/02/16.

[48] Fisher JN, Kitabchi AE. A randomized study of phosphate therapy in the treatment of diabetic ketoacidosis. The Journal of clinical endocrinology and metabolism. 1983;57(1):177-80. Epub 1983/07/01.

[49] Wilson HK, Keuer SP, Lea AS, Boyd AE, 3rd, Eknoyan G. Phosphate therapy in diabetic ketoacidosis. Archives of internal medicine. 1982;142(3):517-20. Epub 1982/03/01.

[50] Rosner EA, Strezlecki KD, Clark JA, Lieh-Lai M. Low Thiamine Levels in Children With Type 1 Diabetes and Diabetic Ketoacidosis: A Pilot Study. Pediatric critical care medicine : a journal of the Society of Critical Care Medicine and the World Federation of Pediatric Intensive and Critical Care Societies. 2014. Epub 2015/01/07.

[51] Dunger DB, Sperling MA, Acerini CL, Bohn DJ, Daneman D, Danne TP, et al. ESPE/LWPES consensus statement on diabetic ketoacidosis in children and adolescents. Archives of disease in childhood. 2004;89(2):188-94. Epub 2004/01/23.

[52] Kumar AR, Kaplowitz PB. Patient age, race and the type of diabetes have an impact on the presenting symptoms, latency before diagnosis and laboratory abnormalities at time of diagnosis of diabetes mellitus in children. Journal of clinical research in pediatric endocrinology. 2009;1(5):227-32. Epub 2009/09/01.

[53] Levy-Marchal C, Papoz L, de Beaufort C, Doutreix J, Froment V, Voirin J, et al. Clinical and laboratory features of type 1 diabetic children at the time of diagnosis. Diabetic medicine : a journal of the British Diabetic Association. 1992;9(3):279-84. Epub 1992/04/01.

[54] Pinkey JH, Bingley PJ, Sawtell PA, Dunger DB, Gale EA. Presentation and progress of childhood diabetes mellitus: a prospective population-based study. The Bart's-Oxford Study Group. Diabetologia. 1994;37(1):70-4. Epub 1994/01/01.

[55] Roche EF, Menon A, Gill D, Hoey H. Clinical presentation of type 1 diabetes. Pediatric diabetes. 2005;6(2):75-8. Epub 2005/06/21.

[56] Wolfsdorf J, Glaser N, Sperling MA, American Diabetes A. Diabetic ketoacidosis in infants, children, and adolescents: A consensus statement from the American Diabetes Association. Diabetes care. 2006;29(5):1150-9. Epub 2006/04/29.

[57] Koves IH, Neutze J, Donath S, Lee W, Werther GA, Barnett P, et al. The accuracy of clinical assessment of dehydration during diabetic ketoacidosis in childhood. Diabetes care. 2004;27(10):2485-7. Epub 2004/09/29.

[58] Edge JA, Roy Y, Bergomi A, Murphy NP, Ford-Adams ME, Ong KK, et al. Conscious level in children with diabetic ketoacidosis is related to severity of acidosis and not to blood glucose concentration. Pediatric diabetes. 2006;7(1):11-5. Epub 2006/02/24.

[59] Wolfsdorf JI, Allgrove J, Craig ME, Edge J, Glaser N, Jain V, et al. Diabetic ketoacidosis and hyperglycemic hyperosmolar state. Pediatric diabetes. 2014;15 Suppl 20:154-79. Epub 2014/07/22.

[60] Adrogue HJ, Eknoyan G, Suki WK. Diabetic ketoacidosis: role of the kidney in the acid-base homeostasis re-evaluated. Kidney international. 1984;25(4):591-8. Epub 1984/04/01.

[61] Weisberg LS. Pseudohyponatremia: a reappraisal. The American journal of medicine. 1989;86(3):315-8. Epub 1989/03/01.

[62] Kebler R, McDonald FD, Cadnapaphornchai P. Dynamic changes in serum phosphorus levels in diabetic ketoacidosis. The American journal of medicine. 1985;79(5): 571-6. Epub 1985/11/01.

[63] Carlotti AP, Bohn D, Jankiewicz N, Kamel KS, Davids MR, Halperin ML. A hyperglycaemic hyperosmolar state in a young child: diagnostic insights from a quantitative analysis. QJM : monthly journal of the Association of Physicians. 2007;100(2): 125-37. Epub 2007/02/06.

[64] Rewers A. Current concepts and controversies in prevention and treatment of diabetic ketoacidosis in children. Current diabetes reports. 2012;12(5):524-32. Epub 2012/08/07.

[65] Clark MG, Dalabih A. Variability of DKA Management Among Pediatric Emergency Room and Critical Care Providers: A Call for More Evidence-Based and Cost-Effective Care? Journal of clinical research in pediatric endocrinology. 2014;6(3):190-1. Epub 2014/09/23.

[66] Harris GD, Fiordalisi I, Yu C. Maintaining normal intracranial pressure in a rabbit model during treatment of severe diabetic ketoacidemia. Life sciences. 1996;59(20): 1695-702. Epub 1996/01/01.

[67] Clements RS, Jr., Blumenthal SA, Morrison AD, Winegrad AI. Increased cerebrospinal-fluid pressure during treatment of diabetic ketosis. Lancet. 1971;2(7726):671-5. Epub 1971/09/25.

[68] Mahoney CP, Vlcek BW, DelAguila M. Risk factors for developing brain herniation during diabetic ketoacidosis. Pediatric neurology. 1999;21(4):721-7. Epub 1999/12/02.

[69] Edge JA, Jakes RW, Roy Y, Hawkins M, Winter D, Ford-Adams ME, et al. The UK case-control study of cerebral oedema complicating diabetic ketoacidosis in children. Diabetologia. 2006;49(9):2002-9. Epub 2006/07/19.

[70] Glaser N, Barnett P, McCaslin I, Nelson D, Trainor J, Louie J, et al. Risk factors for cerebral edema in children with diabetic ketoacidosis. The Pediatric Emergency Medicine Collaborative Research Committee of the American Academy of Pediatrics. The New England journal of medicine. 2001;344(4):264-9. Epub 2001/02/15.

[71] Mel JM, Werther GA. Incidence and outcome of diabetic cerebral oedema in childhood: are there predictors? Journal of paediatrics and child health. 1995;31(1):17-20. Epub 1995/02/01.

[72] Felner EI, White PC. Improving management of diabetic ketoacidosis in children. Pediatrics. 2001;108(3):735-40. Epub 2001/09/05.

[73] Adrogue HJ, Barrero J, Eknoyan G. Salutary effects of modest fluid replacement in the treatment of adults with diabetic ketoacidosis. Use in patients without extreme volume deficit. Jama. 1989;262(15):2108-13. Epub 1989/10/20.

[74] Oh MS, Carroll HJ, Uribarri J. Mechanism of normochloremic and hyperchloremic acidosis in diabetic ketoacidosis. Nephron. 1990;54(1):1-6. Epub 1990/01/01.

[75] Fort P, Waters SM, Lifshitz F. Low-dose insulin infusion in the treatment of diabetic ketoacidosis: bolus versus no bolus. The Journal of pediatrics. 1980;96(1):36-40. Epub 1980/01/01.

[76] Lindsay R, Bolte RG. The use of an insulin bolus in low-dose insulin infusion for pediatric diabetic ketoacidosis. Pediatric emergency care. 1989;5(2):77-9. Epub 1989/06/01.

[77] Kitabchi AE. Low-dose insulin therapy in diabetic ketoacidosis: fact or fiction? Diabetes/metabolism reviews. 1989;5(4):337-63. Epub 1989/06/01.

[78] Nallasamy K, Jayashree M, Singhi S, Bansal A. Low-dose vs standard-dose insulin in pediatric diabetic ketoacidosis: a randomized clinical trial. JAMA pediatrics. 2014;168(11):999-1005. Epub 2014/09/30.

[79] Vincent M, Nobecourt E. Treatment of diabetic ketoacidosis with subcutaneous insulin lispro: a review of the current evidence from clinical studies. Diabetes & metabolism. 2013;39(4):299-305. Epub 2013/05/07.

[80] Barski L, Kezerle L, Zeller L, Zektser M, Jotkowitz A. New approaches to the use of insulin in patients with diabetic ketoacidosis. European journal of internal medicine. 2013;24(3):213-6. Epub 2013/02/12.

[81] Becker DJ, Brown DR, Steranka BH, Drash AL. Phosphate replacement during treatment of diabetic ketosis. Effects on calcium and phosphorus homeostasis. American journal of diseases of children. 1983;137(3):241-6. Epub 1983/03/01.

[82] Zipf WB, Bacon GE, Spencer ML, Kelch RP, Hopwood NJ, Hawker CD. Hypocalcemia, hypomagnesemia, and transient hypoparathyroidism during therapy with potassium phosphate in diabetic ketoacidosis. Diabetes care. 1979;2(3):265-8. Epub 1979/05/01.

[83] Morris LR, Murphy MB, Kitabchi AE. Bicarbonate therapy in severe diabetic ketoacidosis. Annals of internal medicine. 1986;105(6):836-40. Epub 1986/12/01.

[84] Green SM, Rothrock SG, Ho JD, Gallant RD, Borger R, Thomas TL, et al. Failure of adjunctive bicarbonate to improve outcome in severe pediatric diabetic ketoacidosis. Annals of emergency medicine. 1998;31(1):41-8. Epub 1998/01/23.

[85] Hale PJ, Crase J, Nattrass M. Metabolic effects of bicarbonate in the treatment of diabetic ketoacidosis. British medical journal. 1984;289(6451):1035-8. Epub 1984/10/20.

[86] Okuda Y, Adrogue HJ, Field JB, Nohara H, Yamashita K. Counterproductive effects of sodium bicarbonate in diabetic ketoacidosis. The Journal of clinical endocrinology and metabolism. 1996;81(1):314-20. Epub 1996/01/01.

[87] Assal JP, Aoki TT, Manzano FM, Kozak GP. Metabolic effects of sodium bicarbonate in management of diabetic ketoacidosis. Diabetes. 1974;23(5):405-11. Epub 1974/05/01.

[88] Ohman JL, Jr., Marliss EB, Aoki TT, Munichoodappa CS, Khanna VV, Kozak GP. The cerebrospinal fluid in diabetic ketoacidosis. The New England journal of medicine. 1971;284(6):283-90. Epub 1971/02/11.

[89] Glaser N. Cerebral edema in children with diabetic ketoacidosis. Current diabetes reports. 2001;1(1):41-6. Epub 2003/05/24.

[90] Duck SC, Kohler E. Cerebral edema in diabetic ketoacidosis. The Journal of pediatrics. 1981;98(4):674-6. Epub 1981/04/01.

[91] Glaser NS, Wootton-Gorges SL, Marcin JP, Buonocore MH, Dicarlo J, Neely EK, et al. Mechanism of cerebral edema in children with diabetic ketoacidosis. The Journal of pediatrics. 2004;145(2):164-71. Epub 2004/08/04.

[92] Glaser NS, Marcin JP, Wootton-Gorges SL, Buonocore MH, Rewers A, Strain J, et al. Correlation of clinical and biochemical findings with diabetic ketoacidosis-related cerebral edema in children using magnetic resonance diffusion-weighted imaging. The Journal of pediatrics. 2008;153(4):541-6. Epub 2008/07/01.

[93] Vavilala MS, Marro KI, Richards TL, Roberts JS, Curry P, Pihoker C, et al. Change in mean transit time, apparent diffusion coefficient, and cerebral blood volume during pediatric diabetic ketoacidosis treatment. Pediatric critical care medicine : a journal of the Society of Critical Care Medicine and the World Federation of Pediatric Intensive and Critical Care Societies. 2011;12(6):e344-9. Epub 2011/04/26.

[94] Lawrence SE, Cummings EA, Gaboury I, Daneman D. Population-based study of incidence and risk factors for cerebral edema in pediatric diabetic ketoacidosis. The Journal of pediatrics. 2005;146(5):688-92. Epub 2005/05/05.

[95] Watts W, Edge JA. How can cerebral edema during treatment of diabetic ketoacidosis be avoided? Pediatric diabetes. 2014;15(4):271-6. Epub 2014/05/29.

[96] Marcin JP, Glaser N, Barnett P, McCaslin I, Nelson D, Trainor J, et al. Factors associated with adverse outcomes in children with diabetic ketoacidosis-related cerebral edema. The Journal of pediatrics. 2002;141(6):793-7. Epub 2002/12/04.

[97] Paton RC. Haemostatic changes in diabetic coma. Diabetologia. 1981;21(3):172-7. Epub 1981/09/01.

[98] Elding Larsson H, Vehik K, Bell R, Dabelea D, Dolan L, Pihoker C, et al. Reduced prevalence of diabetic ketoacidosis at diagnosis of type 1 diabetes in young children participating in longitudinal follow-up. Diabetes care. 2011;34(11):2347-52. Epub 2011/10/06.

[99] Diabetes Prevention Trial--Type 1 Diabetes Study G. Effects of insulin in relatives of patients with type 1 diabetes mellitus. The New England journal of medicine. 2002;346(22):1685-91. Epub 2002/05/31.

[100] Vanelli M, Chiari G, Lacava S, Iovane B. Campaign for diabetic ketoacidosis prevention still effective 8 years later. Diabetes care. 2007;30(4):e12. Epub 2007/03/30.

[101] Vanelli M, Chiari G, Ghizzoni L, Costi G, Giacalone T, Chiarelli F. Effectiveness of a prevention program for diabetic ketoacidosis in children. An 8-year study in schools and private practices. Diabetes care. 1999;22(1):7-9. Epub 1999/05/20.

[102] King BR, Howard NJ, Verge CF, Jack MM, Govind N, Jameson K, et al. A diabetes awareness campaign prevents diabetic ketoacidosis in children at their initial presentation with type 1 diabetes. Pediatric diabetes. 2012;13(8):647-51. Epub 2012/07/24.

[103] Hoffman WH, O'Neill P, Khoury C, Bernstein SS. Service and education for the insulin-dependent child. Diabetes care. 1978;1(5):285-8. Epub 1978/09/01.

[104] Drozda DJ, Dawson VA, Long DJ, Freson LS, Sperling MA. Assessment of the effect of a comprehensive diabetes management program on hospital admission rates of children with diabetes mellitus. The Diabetes educator. 1990;16(5):389-93. Epub 1990/09/01.

[105] Grey M, Boland EA, Davidson M, Li J, Tamborlane WV. Coping skills training for youth with diabetes mellitus has long-lasting effects on metabolic control and quality of life. The Journal of pediatrics. 2000;137(1):107-13. Epub 2000/07/13.

[106] Beck JK, Logan KJ, Hamm RM, Sproat SM, Musser KM, Everhart PD, et al. Reimbursement for pediatric diabetes intensive case management: a model for chronic diseases? Pediatrics. 2004;113(1 Pt 1):e47-50. Epub 2004/01/02.

[107] Harris MA, Wagner DV, Heywood M, Hoehn D, Bahia H, Spiro K. Youth repeatedly hospitalized for DKA: proof of concept for novel interventions in children's healthcare (NICH). Diabetes care. 2014;37(6):e125-6. Epub 2014/05/24.

[108] Golden MP, Herrold AJ, Orr DP. An approach to prevention of recurrent diabetic ketoacidosis in the pediatric population. The Journal of pediatrics. 1985;107(2):195-200. Epub 1985/08/01.

[109] Laffel LM, Wentzell K, Loughlin C, Tovar A, Moltz K, Brink S. Sick day management using blood 3-hydroxybutyrate (3-OHB) compared with urine ketone monitoring reduces hospital visits in young people with T1DM: a randomized clinical trial. Diabetic medicine : a journal of the British Diabetic Association. 2006;23(3):278-84. Epub 2006/02/24.

Chapter 6

Nutritional Management of Type 1 Diabetes

Shereen Abdelghaffar

Additional information is available at the end of the chapter

http://dx.doi.org/10.5772/61150

Abstract

This chapter focuses on medical nutrition therapy (MNT) in type 1 diabetes mellitus (T1DM), which is vital to achieve metabolic control in patients suffering from this disease. The nutritional goals for people with T1DM are reviewed, which aim at maintaining near-normal blood glucose levels by coordinating insulin therapy, diet, and physical activity patterns. A nutrition prescription is given, and recommendations for appropriate MNT in type 1 diabetes are deduced. Glycemic targets in people with T1DM are highlighted; moreover, the principle of carbohydrate consistency and insulin adjustments with food intake are stressed upon. Meal planning approaches to achieve carbohydrate consistency, including carbohydrate counting, exchange system, and sample meal plans, are explained. Weight management, energy requirements, macronutrients and micronutrients needs, as well as nutritional management during exercise and supports take special attention in this chapter.

Information in this chapter is retrieved from evidence-based resources and evidence-based guidelines. If the latter are not available, information retrieved from high-quality research studies, consensus statements, and well-based experts opinions are included.

Keywords: Medical nutrition therapy, type 1 diabetes mellitus, carbohydrate consistency, meal plans

1. Introduction

Management of type 1 diabetes mellitus (T1DM) is a complex task, integrating multiple factors, but it is ultimately centered on the approach to nutrition. Proper attention to diet is a major factor in minimizing hypoglycemia and weight gain while achieving glycemic control; the latter has been shown to markedly diminish the likelihood of chronic diabetic complications, namely, neuropathy, nephropathy, retinopathy, and coronary artery disease (CAD), in patients with type 1 diabetes [1].

2. General principles of Medical Nutrition Therapy (MNT) in type 1 diabetes

MNT is an integral component of diabetes management and diabetes self-management education. Nutrition advice should be tailored for people with T1DM based on age, medical, lifestyle, and personal factors, taking into account associated diabetes complications and other concomitant conditions for every individual. Consideration should also be given to an individual's culture and beliefs, eating patterns, and food availability [2].

The following aspects should be highly considered:

i. **The nutrition prescription: ABC**

Optimally manage the "ABCs" of diabetes control:

- Glycated hemoglobin (**A**1C)
- **B**lood pressure
- Low-density lipoprotein (LDL)-**c**holesterol

ii. **The nutritional goals for people with type 1 diabetes [3]**

- Maintain blood glucose (BG) concentrations in as physiologically a normal range as possible, by coordinating diet and physical activity patterns and insulin therapy.
- Minimize episodes of hypoglycemia.
- Maintain optimal blood pressure and lipid levels.
- Manage weight appropriately by providing adequate calories, thus also ensuring normal growth and development for children and adolescents with T1DM both physically and emotionally.
- Manage risk factors and prevent complications of diabetes.
- Improve overall health through healthful food choices.
- Address individual nutrition needs, incorporating personal and cultural preferences [3].

iii. **General recommendations for MNT in type 1 diabetes**

Current nutrition recommendations for children and adolescents with diabetes mellitus are rooted in the same principles as those established for all healthy children and adolescents

http://dx.doi.org/10.5772/61150

without diabetes. Individualized meal plans should emphasize a wide variety of healthy food choices to meet the recommended nutrient intakes for essential vitamins and minerals, energy, and fiber and to provide for normal growth and development [4].

The patient should be advised of the following:

- Adhering to the negotiated meal plan
- Adjusting food and/or insulin in response to hyperglycemia
- Adjusting insulin dose for meal size and content
- Appropriately treating hypoglycemia [5]

Glycemic targets in people with diabetes are as follows:

- Fasting BG: 90–130 mg%
- Two-hour postprandial (2 h pp); BG: less than 180 mg%
- Glucose excursion: 2 h pp more than BG before meal by 30–50 mg%
- HBA1c: less than 7 mg% [1]

MNT for type 1diabetes should consider five key aspects:

1. Establishing carbohydrate consistency at meals and snacks
2. Adjusting insulin for variations in blood glucose, food, or physical activity
3. Balancing caloric intake and expenditure for optimum weight management
4. Balancing the nutritional content of selected protein, carbohydrates, and fats
5. Adjusting meal-insulin timing [6]

2.1. Carbohydrate consistency

- Variations in food intake, particularly carbohydrate, should be minimized to avoid fluctuations in blood glucose. Reductions in medication or insulin doses are necessary when there is decrease in carbohydrate intake.
- When using a long-acting basal insulin and a rapid-acting insulin as bolus doses, this allows flexibility in adjustments of insulin dose according to carbohydrate intake. On the other hand, using fixed doses of short- and intermediate-acting insulin require more carbohydrate consistency in timing and amounts.
- Patients who use short-acting insulin analogs or who use insulin pumps may need to take additional bolus insulin injections with snacks that contain more than 10–15 g of carbohydrate [7].

2.2. Meal planning

There are several meal planning approaches to achieve carbohydrate consistency, including [8]

1. carbohydrate counting
2. the exchange system
3. sample meal plans

2.3. Carbohydrate counting

The methods for counting carbohydrate are as follows:

1. **Reading food labels:** looking at the grams of carbohydrates on the label.
2. **Using the exchange system:** estimation of carbohydrate content can be broken down into three food groups that are standardized for carbohydrate content according to particular portions, which are carbohydrate, meat and meat substitutes, and fat. Table1 shows calories and macronutrient content of exchange lists. The exchange lists also identify foods that are good sources of fiber and foods that have high sodium content [9].

Group	Carbohydrate (g)	Protein (g)	Fat (g)	Calories (Cals)
Carbohydrate group				
Starch	15	3	0–1	80
Fruit	15	0	0	60
Milk	15	8	Varies	90–150
Other carbohydrates	15	Varies	Varies	Varies
Nonstarchy vegetables	5	2	0	25
Meat and meat substitutes				
Very lean	0	7	0–1	35
Lean	0	7	3	55
Medium fat	0	7	5	75
High fat	0	7	8	100
Fat group	0	0	5	45

Table 1. Calories and macronutrient content of exchange lists

3. **Use sample meal plans:** These are defined meal menus that specify the time and amounts of food to be eaten at each meal and snack. Dietitians typically tailor the menus to incorporate food preferences and medical nutrition therapy (MNT) goals. Sample menus are created after review of a person's typical food intake; they are best suited for patients who have fairly routine eating habits and who do not eat a wide variety of foods. They also are appropriate for patients who need structured guidance on what to eat [10].

3. Insulin adjustments with food intake

3.1. Advanced carbohydrate counting

At a more advanced level, carbohydrate counting focuses on adjustment of food, insulin, and activity based on patterns from detailed logs. The patient needs to record the time of meals and snacks, the amount and type of food eaten, the amount of carbohydrate consumed, insulin dose, physical activity, and blood glucose results. Patients should first practice eating consistent amounts of carbohydrate at meals and snacks so that baseline insulin requirements can be matched to usual carbohydrate intake using pre- and postprandial blood glucose testing results. When pre- and postprandial blood glucose levels are in the target range, then insulin-to-carbohydrate ratios can be determined as follows [11]:

Insulin-to-carbohydrate ratios

- Divide the number of grams of carbohydrate eaten at the meal by the number of units of premeal insulin (e.g., 45 g carbohydrate divided by 3 units of insulin is a 1:15 ratio). Insulin-to-carbohydrate ratios can vary with time of day and are affected by stress, illness, and variations in physical activity.
- Insulin-to-carbohydrate ratios can also be calculated using the 450–500 rule:

450–500 rule—calculate the insulin-to-carbohydrate ratio as follows:

Regular insulin-to-carbohydrate ratio = 450 divided by total daily dose (TDD) of insulin.

Rapid acting insulin-to-carbohydrate ratio = 500 divided by TDD of insulin.

- Treatment of hypoglycemia: if the patient is hypoglycemic (blood glucose <70 mg/dL), 10–30 g of fast-acting carbohydrate should be taken. Retesting and retreating is mandatory, without overtreatment, till blood glucose rises >70 mg/dL, then the patient resumes the appropriately calculated insulin doses and carbohydrate requirements [12].

3.2. Weight management in T1DM

The relative importance of caloric intake for an individual patient is dependent on several factors, including the following:

- Current weight in relationship to desirable and healthy body weight (BW)
- Fat distribution and waist circumference
- Glycated hemoglobin (A1C)

Lowering caloric intake and inducing weight loss are of major importance for overweight (body mass index [BMI] ≥25–29.9 kg/m^2) and obese (BMI ≥30 kg/m^2) patients with diabetes because the risk of comorbidities associated with excess adipose tissue increases with BMI in these ranges [13].

In children and adolescents, energy needs can be evaluated by tracking weight gain, BMI, and growth patterns on pediatric growth charts from the Centers for Disease Control and Prevention (CDC) or national growth curves [14].

3.3. Weight gain with intensive insulin therapy

Weight gain is a potential adverse effect of intensive insulin therapy and occurs when insulin dosing matches nutritional intake and glycosuria is eliminated.

If A1C is high enough to promote glycosuria, then lowering calorie intake by an additional 250–300 calories per day is necessary to prevent weight gain with intensification of diabetes therapy. Other strategies to minimize weight gain with intensive therapy are to reduce insulin doses preferentially for patterns of hypoglycemia rather than increasing meal size or adding an undesired snack. To reduce calories further, it is helpful to reduce fat intake and try to keep carbohydrate intake consistent to minimize risk of hypoglycemia [15].

3.4. Total energy expenditure

Easiest way to calculate: 20–35 Cal/kg current weight/day

If the patient's current weight is more than 30% of his ideal BW, it is better to use adjusted BW (ABW)

- ABW = (current BW – ideal BW) × 0.25 + ideal BW

4. Estimating caloric needs to promote weight loss

If 500–1000 calories are subtracted from weight maintenance calories every day, this would lead to loss of 1–2 pounds per week. Low-calorie diets (less than 1200 kcal/day) should be avoided to be sure that nutritional needs are met [16]

4.1. Nutritional content in T1DM

- The optimal macronutrient composition of the diet for patients with diabetes is controversial.
- The mix of dietary carbohydrate, protein, and fat may be adjusted to meet the metabolic goals and individual preferences of the person with T1DM, but in general, daily energy intake should be targeted to include 50–55% carbohydrate, 10–15% protein, and 30–35% fat [3].
- Low-fat, low-carbohydrate, Mediterranean, and vegetarian diet are all acceptable.
- Individualized meal planning should include optimization of food choices to meet the recommended daily allowance (RDA)/dietary reference intake (DRI) for all micronutrients [3]

4.2. Carbohydrates (CHO)

- The RDA/DRI is 60 g for infants 0–6 months, 95 g for infants 7–12 months, and 130 g for children and adolescents. Diets containing less than 130 g of CHO for children older than 1 year may not provide adequate glucose as fuel for the central nervous system without relying on gluconeogenesis from ingested protein and fat. Low-carbohydrate diets also restrict intake of essential nutrients, energy, and fiber from carbohydrates found in whole

http://dx.doi.org/10.5772/61150

grains, fruits, vegetables, dried peas and beans, legumes, nuts and seeds, and low-fat milk and yogurt.

- Monitoring carbohydrate, whether by carbohydrate counting, a choice, or experience-based estimation, remains a key strategy in achieving glycemic control. Monitoring carbohydrate intake is important as it directly determines postprandial blood sugar, and consequent insulin adjustment can improve glycemic control [16].
- For individuals with diabetes, the use of glycemic index and glycemic load may provide a modest additional benefit for glycemic control over that observed when total carbohydrate is considered alone. Meals with low glycemic index and glycemic load leads to better glycemic control.
- Carbohydrates from fruits, vegetables, whole grains, legumes, and low-fat milk are preferable.
- Nonnutritive sweeteners are safe when consumed within daily levels established by the US Food and Drug Administration (FDA). Consumption of nonnutritive sweeteners does not increase blood glucose concentrations or affect insulin response in adults, although no similar data are available in children. When calculating carbohydrate content of foods, one-half of the sugar alcohol content should be counted in the total carbohydrate content of the food. Careful reading of food labels is always recommended for foods containing nonnutritive sweeteners as they still contain carbohydrates [17].

4.3. Sucrose

- Intake of sucrose does not need to be restricted, although care should be taken to avoid excess calories; sucrose can be substituted for other carbohydrate sources in the meal plan or, if added, covered with insulin. Sucrose-containing foods typically provide additional calories from fats and are frequently devoid of essential nutrients. Nutrition therapy strategies should focus on consuming these foods in moderation in the context of a healthy well balanced diet. Use of added fructose as a sweetener is not recommended, as it may adversely affect lipids, but there is no need to avoid fructose occurring naturally in fruits and vegetables [18].

4.4. Fats

- Because of the increased risk of cardiovascular disease in people with T1 DM, nutrition therapy also emphasizes a diet low in *saturated fat*, as outlined by the National Cholesterol Education Program and the American Heart association, for all children and adolescents. Saturated fat intake should be less than 7% of total calories. Saturated fats (eg, in fatty and processed meats, butter, lard, hydrogenated fats, coconut and palm oils, cheese, ice cream, and other high-fat dairy products) can be replaced with monounsaturated (about 20%) and polyunsaturated fatty acids (eg, in fish, olive oil, nuts) (about 10%) due to their relatively cardioprotective profile. Sources include olive, canola and peanut oils; olives; nuts; seeds; and avocados.

- Reducing intakes of trans-fatty acids lowers low-density lipoprotein and increases high-density lipoprotein; therefore, intake of trans-fatty acids should be minimized. Added trans-fatty acids are found in margarine and processed and commercially prepared foods. Total cholesterol should be less than 200 mg daily. Dietary cholesterol is only found in foods of animal origin.
- Omega 3 fatty acids, specifically eicosapentaenoic acid (EPA) and docosahexaenoic acid (DHA), have emerged as important dietary adjuncts for individuals at risk of cardiovascular disease and in adults who have already experienced a cardiovascular event. The American Heart Association currently recommends marine-derived omega-3 fatty acids as a dietary adjunct to aid in reduction of serum triglycerides, which can safely be used in children with diabetes and hypertriglyceridemia. Eating two or more servings of fish per week is recommended to provide an excellent source of omega-3 fatty acids. Other potent sources are salmon, tuna, herring, sardines, mackerel, flax seeds and oil, various nuts, and canola and soybean oil [19].

4.5. Proteins

- In individuals with normal renal function, protein intake is based on the RDA for all children and adolescents. The usual daily intake of protein should be approximately 10–25% of total caloric intake (1.1 gm/kg/d).
- Patients should be encouraged to substitute lean meats, fish, eggs, beans, peas, soy products, low-fat dairy products, legumes and nuts, and seeds for red meat.
- Protein intake should not be used to treat hypoglycemia or prevent hypoglycemia overnight.
- In patients with microalbuminuria, a reduction of protein to 0.8–1 g/kg/d of body weight may slow the progression of nephropathy. Overt nephropathy necessitates reduction of protein to 0.8 g/kg/d [20].

4.6. Fiber

- Fiber intake should be at least 14 g per 1000 calories daily, or approximately 19–38 g of fiber/day. High-fiber diets have been demonstrated to decrease postprandial glucose concentrations among adolescents with T1DM. Dietary fiber is found in whole grains, fruits, vegetables, dried peas, beans, legumes, nuts, and seeds. Soluble fiber sources should be emphasized because studies in people without diabetes show that diets high in total and soluble fiber (7–13 g) can reduce total cholesterol by 2–3% and LDL cholesterol up to 7%. Potent sources of soluble fiber include oatmeal, oat cereal, lentils, apples, oranges, pears, oat bran, strawberries, nuts, flaxseeds, beans, dried peas, blueberries, cucumbers, celery, and carrots [21].

4.7. Sodium

- A reduced sodium intake of 2300 mg per day is advised, which is the same for healthy children and adolescents. However, for individuals with hypertension, further reduction to 1500 mg/day is recommended.

- Avoidance of processed foods, restaurant and fast foods, and soda beverages and preparations containing preservatives is advisable due to high content of sodium [19].

4.8. Micronutrients

- Routine supplementation with antioxidants, such as vitamins E and C and beta-carotene, is not advised because of lack of evidence of efficacy and concerns related to long term safety.
- Low serum 25-hydroxyvitamin D concentrations are globally associated with children and adolescents with T1DM. Vitamin D screening and supplementation should therefore be considered and should be meeting the RDA of 600 IU vitamin D per day.
- Supplementation with vitamins and micronutrients in general is not necessary if a well-balanced, healthy diet is consumed unless there are underlying deficiencies [21].

5. Glycemic index

A food's GI is a numeric value that reflects its glycemic response in comparison to that of a reference food, such as pure glucose. The GI of the reference food is set at 100. When glucose is used as a reference food, foods with GI>70 are considered high-glycemic index, while Foods with GI<55 are considered low-glycemic index. Some examples of low-glycemic index foods include nonstarchy vegetables, nuts, legumes, and certain grains such as barley and converted rice. High glycemic index foods include potatoes, candies, white bread, and other refined products made from grains [22].

6. Glycemic load

Glycemic load is the product of the glycemic index value of a food and its total carbohydrate content. The concept of the glycemic load was developed because the blood glucose response is influenced not only by the quality of the carbohydrate consumed (i.e., the glycemic index) but also by the quantity of carbohydrate consumed.

The glycemic index and glycemic load may have far greater health implications than glycemic control alone. Several prospective studies have associated diets high in glycemic index and glycemic load with an increased risk of developing type 2 diabetes, coronary heart disease, and some cancers. Data also suggest that low-glycemic load diets are particularly effective among the most susceptible individuals, those who are already overweight and insulin resistant [22].

7. Eating disorders

Eating disorders are relatively common in patients with diabetes, especially in female adolescents and young adults with diabetes. Dieting or omission of insulin for weight loss and binge eating are the most common. Eating disorders have a deleterious impact on glycemic control and on long-term outcome in these patients. It is important to evaluate patients with diabetes, especially young women, for an eating disorder (or misreporting of insulin administration) and arrange appropriate psychological and nutritional counseling and support when indicated [23,24].

8. Promoting dietary compliance

- Gradual behavioral and dietary changes should be advised to move the patient toward a more ideal diet and eating pattern.
- The patient's own food records and motivation to learn can be helpful in guiding decisions for meal planning approaches
- Motivating a patient to make a long-term commitment to dietary alterations is a challenge. Achieving and maintaining weight reduction is difficult in any obese patient. Compliance can occasionally be enhanced by the rapid and often dramatic improvements in glycemic control.
- Diabetes Education Workshops for small groups of patients is highly effective.
- Exercise can increase the degree of weight loss, and the likelihood that it will be maintained.
- Offering varieties of lists of meal plans is very helpful
- Adjustment of diet, exercise, and insulin doses according to the patient's changing lifestyle patterns is mandatory to maintain glycemic control and prevent acute and chronic complications [1,25-27].

9. Physical activity in patients with T1DM

Exercise is a significant component of diabetes management [28,29].

9.1. Benefits of exercise

- Improved glycemic control
- Weight control
- Reduction in comorbidities (hypertension, dyslipidemia, and cardiovascular disease)
- Improved mood and quality of life

http://dx.doi.org/10.5772/61150

9.2. General tips for physical activity in T1DM

- Patients with T1DM should engage in 30 min or more of moderate intensity physical activity on most days of the week. Individuals for whom weight loss and weight maintenance are a concern, may need 60–90 min of moderate to vigorous intensity activity 3 days a week.
- For patients who are trying to lose weight, it is preferable to adjust insulin doses rather than increase food intake to compensate for exercise.
- Timing of exercise in relation to insulin dose, type, mode of delivery, and time of injection should be considered.
- Patients with diabetes should check blood sugar levels before and after exercising, especially in the beginning of an exercise program, to evaluate glycemic response to exercise and adjust insulin regimen [28, 29].

9.3. Diabetes and sports

Athletes need additional blood glucose testing prior to exercise, during exercise (especially exercise lasting greater than 60 min), immediately after exercise, several hours after exercise, and at any time significant changes in intensity, type, or duration of exercise are made. If blood glucose is less than 100 mg/dL, CHO intake of 15–40 mg is important before exercise. If blood glucose is high, urine ketones should be tested and exercise prevented until ketones disappear by insulin and medication adjustments. In absence of ketones, exercise with caution can be allowed [28, 29].

9.4. General nutritional tips for performance of sports in T1DM

- Preactivity meals (1–2 h before exercise) should be relatively high in carbohydrate, moderate to high in protein and low in fat.
- Protein of high biological value (1 gram of protein per pound of body weight) should be used.
- Protein shake can be used before workout (a shake containing at least 6 g of amino acids—the muscle-building blocks of protein—and 35 g of carbohydrates 30–60 min before exercising increases protein synthesis more than drinking the same shake after training.
- Good-quality whey-protein powders usually contain at least 30 g of protein per serving, as well as a healthy supply of vitamins and minerals.
- Weight-gain powders can also provide a lot of high-quality protein and nutrients in each serving, but they also tend to be extremely high in calories, carbohydrates, and sugar.
- Vigorous exercise involving a muscle group shortly after having injected insulin near to that area could cause the insulin to be absorbed more rapidly than usual, increasing the chances of hypoglycemia.
- Competitive/power exercise can lead to hyperglycemia.

- Individual reactions may vary, and so it is best to verify this by checking blood glucose levels before the burst of activity and about 30 min after, to see how the body responds.
- Warming up is necessary to reduce injury

9.5. During exercise

- During exercise lasting more than 30 min, 15–30 gm CHO should be consumed every 30–60 min.
- Sport drinks, dilute juices, sport bars, and/or high fiber cookies should be carried in a food bag to be consumed during exercise.
- Keeping hydrated by drinking around 150 ml of fluid every 15 min is advised.
- CHO foods should be available during and after exercise.

9.6. After exercise

- After a period of strenuous activity or a long period of exercise, blood sugar levels can drop for up to 48 h. Management includes reducing insulin requirements or dosage of antidiabetic drugs over this period, or take more carbohydrate.
- A high-quality protein meal should be consumed after training.
- Omega-3 fatty acids are beneficial.
- Rest: a full-body workout should be followed by a day of rest or alternatively, at least 3 days of rest each week is advised [28, 29].

10. Summary and conclusion

Achieving metabolic control in patients with T1DM cannot be reached except with proper medical nutrition therapy. Nutrition advice should be customized according to age, medical condition, lifestyle, and personal factors. The nutritional goals for people with type 1 diabetes are to maintain blood glucose (BG) concentrations in a physiologically normal range as possible, by coordinating diet and physical activity patterns and insulin therapy, minimizing episodes of hypoglycemia, maintaining optimal blood pressure and lipid levels, and managing weight appropriately, and by providing adequate calories, thus also ensuring normal growth and development for children and adolescents with T1DM both physically and emotionally. Although a focus on careful carbohydrate counting is integral to insulin delivery and glycemic control for patients with T1DM, many of the other fundamental principles of nutrition management are important to be considered. The patient should be advised for adhering to the negotiated meal plan, adjusting food and/or insulin in response to hyperglycemia, as well as adjusting insulin dose for meal size and content and appropriately treating hypoglycemia. Proper estimation of energy requirements, macronutrients, and micronutrients needs as well as adjustment of MNT during exercise and sports are all of high importance. A team approach,

http://dx.doi.org/10.5772/61150

capitalizing on the expertise of pediatric and adult dietitians, psychologists, nurses, and physicians, can best assist patients and their families overcome challenges in their care and reach their therapeutic goals.

Author details

Shereen Abdelghaffar*

Address all correspondence to: sh.abdelghaffar@gmail.com

Pediatric Diabetes and Endocrinology Cairo University, Egypt

References

[1] American Academy of Pediatrics. Pediatric Nutrition. Nutrition Therapy for Children and Adolescents with Type 1 and 2 Diabetes Mellitus. 7th edition. Chapter 31. 2013 pp 741–769

[2] Franz MJ, Bantle JP, Beebe CA, et al. Evidence-based nutrition principles and recommendations for the treatment and prevention of diabetes and related complications. Diabetes Care 2002; 25:148.

[3] American Diabetes Association. Standards of medical care in diabetes—2014. Diabetes Care 2014; 37 Suppl 1:S14.

[4] Anderson EJ, Richardson M, Castle G, et al. Nutrition interventions for intensive therapy in the Diabetes Control and Complications Trial. The DCCT Research Group. Journal of the American Dietetic Association 1993; 93:768.

[5] Brand-Miller J, Hayne S, Petocz P, Colagiuri S. Low-glycemic index diets in the management of diabetes: a meta-analysis of randomized controlled trials. Diabetes Care 2003; 26:2261.

[6] Buyken AE, Toeller M, Heitkamp G, et al. Glycemic index in the diet of European outpatients with type 1 diabetes: relations to glycated hemoglobin and serum lipids. American Journal of Clinical Nutrition 2001; 73:574.

[7] Close EJ, Wiles PG, Lockton JA, et al. The degree of day-to-day variation in food intake in diabetic patients. Diabetic Medicine 1993; 10:514.

[8] Delahanty LM, Halford BN. The role of diet behaviors in achieving improved glycemic control in intensively treated patients in the Diabetes Control and Complications Trial. Diabetes Care 1993; 16:1453.

[9] Delahanty L, Simkins SW, Camelon K. Expanded role of the dietitian in the Diabetes Control and Complications Trial: implications for clinical practice. The DCCT Research Group. J Am Diet Assoc 1993; 93:758.

[10] Delahanty LM, Nathan DM, Lachin JM, et al. Association of diet with glycated hemoglobin during intensive treatment of type 1 diabetes in the Diabetes Control and Complications Trial. American Journal of Clinical Nutrition 2009; 89:518.

[11] Dumesnil JG, Turgeon J, Tremblay A, et al. Effect of a low-glycaemic index–low-fat–high protein diet on the atherogenic metabolic risk profile of abdominally obese men. British Journal of Nutrition 2001; 86:557.

[12] Evert AB, Boucher JL, Cypress M, et al. Nutrition therapy recommendations for the management of adults with diabetes. Diabetes Care 2013; 36:3821.

[13] Franz MJ. Finding the right fit for meal planning. Diabetes Care 1993; 16:1043.

[14] Centers for Disease Control and Prevention. Clinical Growth Chart. Available at: http://www.cdc.gov/growth charts/clinical_charts.htm. Accessed December 2014.

[15] Heller SR, Clarke P, Daly H, et al. Group education for obese patients with type 2 diabetes: greater success at less cost. Diabetic Med 1988; 5:552.

[16] Jenkins DJ, Wolever TM, Taylor RH, et al. Glycemic index of foods: a physiological basis for carbohydrate exchange. American Journal of Clinical Nutrition 1981; 34:362.

[17] Johnston CS, Buller AJ. Vinegar and peanut products as complementary foods to reduce postprandial glycemia. Journal of the American Dietetic Association 2005; 105:1939.

[18] Mannucci E, Rotella F, Ricca V, et al. Eating disorders in patients with type 1 diabetes: a meta-analysis. Journal of Endocrinological Investication 2005; 28:417.

[19] Nathan DM, Cleary PA, Backlund JY, et al. Intensive diabetes treatment and cardiovascular disease in patients with type 1 diabetes. New England Journal of Medicine 2005; 353:2643.

[20] Nuttall FQ. Carbohydrate and dietary management of individuals with insulin-requiring diabetes. Diabetes Care 1993; 16:1039.

[21] Pastors JG, Waslaski J, Gunderson H. Diabetes meal-planning strategies. In: Diabetes Medical Nutrition Therapy and Education, Ross TA, Boucher JL, O'Connell BS (Eds.), American Diabetes Association, Chicago, IL; 2005.

[22] Wolever TM, Nguyen PM, Chiasson JL, et al. Determinants of diet glycemic index calculated retrospectively from diet records of 342 individuals with noninsulin-dependent diabetes mellitus. American Journal of Clinical Nutrition 1994; 59:1265.

[23] Peveler RC, Bryden KS, Neil HA, et al. The relationship of disordered eating habits citand attitudes to clinical outcomes in young adult females with type 1 diabetes. Diabetes Care 2005; 28:84.

[24] Rabasa-Lhoret R, Garon J, Langelier H, et al. Effects of meal carbohydrate content on insulin requirements in type 1 diabetic patients treated intensively with the basal-bolus (ultralente-regular) insulin regimen. Diabetes Care 1999; 22:667.

[25] Rydall AC, Rodin GM, Olmsted MP, et al. Disordered eating behavior and microvascular complications in young women with insulin-dependent diabetes mellitus. New England Journal of Medicine 1997; 336:1849.

[26] Wolever TM. Carbohydrate and the regulation of blood glucose and metabolism. Nutr Rev 2003; 61:S40.

[27] Wolever TM, Hamad S, Chiasson JL, et al. Day-to-day consistency in amount and source of carbohydrate intake associated with improved blood glucose control in type 1 diabetes. Journal of the American College of Nursing 1999; 18:242.

[28] American Diabetes Association. Physical activity/exercise and diabetes. Diabetes Care 2004; 27 Suppl 1:S58.

[29] Brooks GA, Butte NF, Rand WM, et al. Chronicle of the Institute of Medicine physical activity recommendation: how a physical activity recommendation came to be among dietary recommendations. American Journal of Clinical Nutrition 2004; 79:921S.

Chapter 7

The Role of Family Functioning on Metabolic Control and Quality of Life in Adolescents with Type 1 Diabetes Mellitus

Ana Cristina Almeida, Engrácia Leandro and Maria da Graça Pereira

Additional information is available at the end of the chapter

http://dx.doi.org/10.5772/60732

Abstract

The incidence of type 1 diabetes mellitus (T1DM) in childhood and adolescents is increasing worldwide and diagnosis of type 1 diabetes represents an important stressful condition for families and adolescents. The maintenance of normal glycemic results requires adherence to self-care behaviors in order to prevent disease complications. However, diabetes self-care requires extensive and daily behavioral demands from adolescents that may interfere with their quality of life.

Parents have an important influence on T1DM' management, in adolescents. Family functioning is an important determinant of metabolic control and adolescents' quality of life. During adolescence, parents must transfer the responsibility for diabetes care to the adolescent and supervise diabetes management. Parental style and family conflict are related to glycemic control and quality of life in adolescents.

The main goal of this chapter was to analyze the relationship between metabolic control, quality of life and family functioning in T1DM adolescents.

Keywords: Metabolic Control, Quality of Life, Family Functioning, Type 1 Diabetes, Adolescents

1. Introduction

T1DM is one of the most common chronic illnesses in children and adolescents [1, 2]. This chronic disease and its serious complications forces both adolescents and families into an abrupt lifestyle change and psychosocial adjustment [3]. An intensive daily glycemic control and treatment regimen have been associated with a better control of the disease, reduced complications and improved quality of life [3, 4]. T1DM self-management activities include metabolic control monitoring at least four times a day, frequent insulin injections (at least four times a day), adjustment of insulin doses to match carbohydrate intake and engagement in physical activities [1, 5]. Management of T1DM requires changes in the lifestyle of both the adolescent and his/her family, which can contribute to distress and diminished quality of life of both adolescents with diabetes and parents [6].

T1DM occurs when pancreatic β cells cannot produce insulin due to an autoimmune process which destroys these cells. The conversion of food into energy is abruptly interrupted, requiring an insulin therapeutic regimen to meet a person's need for insulin [3, 7].

In adolescence, individuals are confronted with biological, physical and psychosocial changes which indirectly affect their levels of glycosylated hemoglobin which tend to be high due to both the hormonal components of puberty and the transfer of responsibility for diabetes management from parents to adolescents [7, 8]. Adolescents with T1DM have been found to have worse metabolic control than individuals of other age groups which is associated with an increased risk of developing diabetes complications [9]. Adolescents play an ever-increasing role in diabetes management, according to their developmental acquisitions [5, 10]. However, adolescents' risk behaviors, such as those related with their sexual development, use of illicit drugs, smoking and alcohol, and the vulnerability to the development of mental health problems also compromise their metabolic and psychological outcomes [3, 5]. In the transition to adolescence, young people with T1DM tend to have poor self-management, which deteriorates metabolic control, increases psychosocial distress and negatively influences their quality of life [11]. The stress caused by the feeling of being different from their peers, as a result, of self-management activities which disrupt their daily activities, and the sense of guilt, over exhibiting poor metabolic results, may negatively impact adolescents' quality of life [12, 13].

The presence of a chronic illness during adolescence not only affects the adolescent, but also interferes with family functioning. Nevertheless, family also influences illness outcomes due to their communication patterns, interaction styles and problem-solving skills [14].

While building upon the model of childhood adaptation to T1DM [15], the aim of this study is to describe the relationship between family functioning, metabolic control and quality of life, in T1DM adolescents.

2. Adolescents with T1DM:: The process of adaptation

In adolescence, the experience of new cognitive and psychosocial competences and independence desires, by the adolescents, interferes with the relationship with their parents. This may influence adolescents' performance regarding diabetes management and, consequently, adolescents' process of adaptation to the illness itself [16].

As Butner and colleagues [16] point out in their study on the parent-adolescent's discrepancies with respect to diabetes management, adolescents tend to perceive themselves as more competent and independent than parents. This situation has an impact on the daily family diabetes activities and on the well-being of both parents and adolescents leading often to conflicts, conflicts, poorer metabolic control, well-being and, consequently, poorer illness adjustment.

The adaptation process to T1DM is complex for both adolescents and their families, and requires time and effort with regard to the daily treatment regimen [17]. The internal and external factors that influence the physiological and psychological adaptation process of T1DM adolescents have been largely recognized in literature and have been identified in theoretical childhood adaptation models ino T1DM [6].

The Childhood Adaptation Model to Chronic Illness: Diabetes Mellitus [15] identifies factors that influence childhood adaptation to T1DM and posits that individual and family characteristics such as age, socioeconomic status, race/ethnicity, treatment modality, individuals' and families' responses – like self-management, coping, self-efficacy, family functioning and social competence – influence metabolic control and the quality of life of adolescents with T1DM, i.e., level of adaptation. The model allows the identification of modifiable risk and protective factors, in the adjustment process of adolescents with T1DM [15]. According to the Childhood Adaptation Model, metabolic control and quality of life of T1DM adolescents are considered key factors in the adaptation process to diabetes, and a good adaptation is dependent on good glycemic levels and a positive quality of life [5, 6]. Family functioning is considered a potential mediator of the stress felt by the children and their parents, caused by the presence of a chronic disease, and the family and child adaptation process to diabetes [15].

3. Metabolic control in adolescents with diabetes

Metabolic control is recognized as the most important marker of physiological adaptation to T1DM, but adolescents with this disease tend to show some difficulty in achieving it [7]. Optimal glycemic levels require the balance of dietary intake, physical activity and the adjustment of insulin doses [18, 19]. For T1DM adolescents, the American Diabetes Association (ADA) [20] recommends maintaining hemoglobin A1C values below 7.5% to prevent and delay medical complications, such as microvascular and neuropathic complications [20]. However, the metabolic control of T1DM adolescents presents suboptimal results (range from 7.5% to 9%) [21] which tend to increase the adolescent and the family stress levels, because they feel unable to achieve and maintain normal glycemic levels to prevent hypoglycemic episodes and long-term complications [22].

Metabolic control is measured by glycated hemoglobin, which represents the average over the last 2–3 months of blood glucose and is internationally recognized as the standard measure of metabolic control [7].

Individual factors such as pubertal development, disease duration and race/ethnicity, affect metabolic control of T1DM adolescents with type 1 diabetes [7]. Literature has suggested that longer diabetes duration and pubertal development are linked to poor metabolic control in adolescents with diabetes [7]. During puberty, the decrease in insulin sensibility caused by growth hormone results in poor metabolic control among of T1DM [11]. Also, problem-solving skills of immature adolescents, and rebellion against parents' participation in diabetes management are linked to poor metabolic control [23].

However, metabolic control tends to deteriorate during puberty due to the independence and autonomy from parent's orientation in diabetes self-management and behavior changes during adolescence [7]. If parents continue to encourage their children to participate in their diabetes care during adolescence and participate in their children's diabetes treatments, adolescents will have better glycemic and psychosocial results [22]. Also, the level and type of parent involvement in adolescents' diabetes management must change according to the adolescent developmental stage to avoid family conflicts and consequently a negative impact on adolescents' metabolic control and quality of life [24, 25].

Regarding the role of metabolic control in the adaptation process of adolescents with diabetes and, according to the study of Malik and Koot [10], metabolic control was a predictor of the adjustment of adolescents to T1DM; however, the small explained variance in adolescent adjustment was interpreted as metabolic control having little influence on adolescent's adjustment to diabetes.

The association between metabolic control and quality of life in T1DM adolescents is controversial [26]. While some studies have found a link between higher metabolic control and lower well-being [27, 28], others did not find any relationship between metabolic control and quality of life, in T1DM adolescents [9, 29]. Literature has suggested that metabolic control was improved in adolescents who reported good quality of life, and who were supported by a stable and cohesive family with a clear defined sharing responsibility, in diabetes management [21].

4. Adolescents' quality of life and T1DM

Quality of life is recognized as one important psychosocial outcome in adolescents with diabetes [17]. The individual subjective experience of the impact caused by the illness and its treatment, on the physical, psychosocial and cultural domains of one´s individual performance defines health-related quality of life [30]. The frequent measure of quality of life in T1DM adolescents is useful to understand how they cope with diabetes tasks and how they include care in their daily activities [30]. Moreover, in the monitoring of quality of life of adolescents, it is important to consider how the type of diabetes treatment, the diabetes symptoms, the social and emotional development of adolescents, and the adolescents' academic performance influences their quality of life [31].

T1DM adolescents tend to report good quality of life despite the complex process of disease management [29]. Quality of life in T1DM adolescents is also similar to the quality of life levels of healthy adolescents, in spite of their parents´ perceptions [9, 31]. However, the diabetes burden on routine activities and their impact on relationship with friends, interfere with emotional and social well-being of adolescents with diabetes, which may negatively affect the adolescent's quality of life [9, 13]. In their longitudinal study with Chinese adolescents with T1DM, Guo and colleagues [32] found a positive association between self-management care and satisfaction with quality of life. This fact may be explained by family support and self-efficacy influence in the relationship between self-care management and satisfaction with quality of life [17]. Kalyva, Malakonaki, Eiser and Mamoulakis [13] concluded that quality of life was better, in male adolescents with better glycemic control, shorter duration of diabetes and younger age at diabetes onset. In the same study, it was found that older adolescents reported better quality of life when compared with younger adolescents, and this result may be explained by the fact that older adolescents have more autonomy, in their diabetes management. Guo et al. [17] also found that diabetes duration had an impact on adolescents' quality of life, with less duration of diabetes predicting better quality of life. These findingss may be explained by the dominant influence of parents on the adolescents' diabetes management [17].

The literature has suggested that metabolic control is a significant predictor of the adolescent quality of life [10], is associated with adolescent's adjustment to T1DM, and that quality of life of adolescents with diabetes is related to family support [33].

Literature has suggested that higher quality of life was related to better metabolic control in adolescents [21]. However, in adolescents with diabetes, quality of life may not be related to metabolic control, if soon after the onset of diabetes, adolescents and their families were integrated in intervention programs to develop and increase their ability to diabetes management [31].

In order to analyze the better quality of life successful prevention interventions in T1DM adolescents, Fogel and Weiss-Benchell [30] observed that some interventions, such as education sessions or motivational interviewing, improved quality of life in adolescents with diabetes, but without the concomitant results in their levels of glycemic control, which may explain the special relationship between quality of life and metabolic control, in T1DM adolescents.

5. Family functioning: The relationship with metabolic control and quality of life

In the complex process of diabetes self-management, adolescents and their families share the responsibility and decision-making process in the illness-related activities to achieve the goals of diabetes control and well-being [7]. Family functioning represents an important factor in the diabetes management treatment in T1DM adolescents and affecting metabolic control and quality of life outcomes [27, 34]. The study of Skinner, John and Hampson [35], that studied the relationship between family factors and metabolic control, including family functioning, concluded that family factors were predictors of metabolic control, accounting for 34% of the variance in metabolic control.

Table 1 shows some of the most important parental strategies to improve better metabolic control and quality of life in T1DM adolescents.

Parental Strategies to Improve Metabolic Control and Quality of Life in Adolescents with T1DM
• Negotiation of parental supervision regarding adolescents' diabetes management (food intake, glycemic control, adjustment of insulin doses and exercise);
• Parental supervision of adolescent diabetes care, according to the developmental adolescence stage;
• Gradually transfer diabetes care responsibility to adolescents when they demonstrated the adequate skills to deal with diabetes care tasks;
• Support emotionally the adolescents when they felt unable to achieve and maintain normal glycemic levels;
• Clear definition of the shared responsibility between parents and adolescents about diabetes management, to avoid parental overinvolvement;
• Development of a collaborative family organization characterized by guidance and supervision from parents;
• Clear and warm communication patterns between parents and adolescents related to adolescent diabetes care;
• Development of skills to deal with the stress caused by diabetes care;
• Development of stable, supportive and cohesive family interaction with adolescents;
• Emotional support and positive reinforcement of successful adolescents' diabetes management;
• Avoid negative parenting behaviors such as hostility and conflicts about adolescents' diabetes management.

Table 1. Parents strategies to promote better metabolic control and quality of life in adolescents with type 1 diabetes

Literature has suggested that family functioning was strongly associated with better metabolic control, psychosocial functioning and psychological adjustment in T1DM children and adolescents with type 1 diabetes [36]. Parents of children with diabetes, particularly mothers, tend to experience greater levels of psychosocial distress and adjustment problems due to the responsibility required by diabetes management on daily family activities [1]. Studies have demonstrated that higher family anxiety and less positive parenting strategies are linked to negative family perception about adolescent's self-management, which may exacerbate adolescents' neglected self-care and compromise their glycemic results [3]. Psychological adjustment problems in mothers of children with diabetes have been related to poorer psychological adjustment and higher levels of distress in T1DM children [37]. Other studies have found that negative family functioning increased conflicts between parents and children affecting negatively the child metabolic control, especially in older children [35]. Children's developmental process with the acquisition of more competences and independence, regarding diabetes care, may be related with the maturation process of puberty [16, 35]. Pertaining to what may originate family conflict between T1DM adolescents and their parents, Fogel and Weissberg-Benchell [30] mentioned conflicts caused by what adolescents think they hear from their parents (nagging and criticism) when parents try to express worry and concern with the adolescent's disease.

Family factors were related to adolescents' metabolic control [7, 35] and quality of life [9]. Whilst, in one research about family influence on adolescents' diabetes outcome, higher conflict between parents and adolescents were associated with poor metabolic control [34,

35], in another study, better family structure and positive parental emotional support were related to better metabolic control in T1DM adolescents [36, 38].

Although during adolescence, parents must transfer the responsibility for diabetes management into the adolescents, the literature has shown how parental monitoring and family support influence health outcomes in T1DM adolescents, in spite of their desire for independence and autonomy [34]. Literature has suggested that older adolescents have more risk to neglect diabetes self-management than younger adolescents, which makes parental involvement more crucial during adolescence [39].

However, the quality of parental support and monitoring is crucial, because when adolescents perceive that parents are overinvolved in their diabetes care and consider parents' guidance and control being too much, metabolic control tends to be negatively influenced [34, 40]. Also, Skinner, John and Hampson [35] observed that adolescents who perceived the relationship with parents more critical, unsupportive and negative regarding their diabetes management, showed worse metabolic control. Therefore, research advocates a collaborative family style, characterized by an appropriated guidance and control from parents, to improve metabolic control and quality of life in T1DM adolescents, and consequently a better diabetes adaptation [22, 35, 41]. When Faulkner and Chang [18] interviewed adolescents and their parents about what promoted better adolescents' performance, in their diabetes management, the results showed that a directive guidance (be an aid to perform) and tangible (physical) assistance were considered as being useful in improving metabolic results, in adolescents. Also family environment, characterized by warm, caring, and cohesive interactions between adolescents and parents, was related to better self-management, glycemic control and quality of life in young T1DM adolescents [18, 33]. In their study about observed parenting in T1DM adolescents and their mothers, Jaser and Grey [36] concluded that sensitive parenting behaviors and child-centered and positive reinforcement were related to better illness adaptation and better metabolic control, while maternal hostility, considered as negative parenting behaviors, was associated with worse metabolic control in adolescents. Also Monaghan and colleagues [42], in their study about the relationship between parents' stress, parenting style and self-care in T1DM pre-adolescents, concluded that greater parental warmth and flexibility were related to less parenting stress related to diabetes care, which contributed to the decrease of family conflict and, consequently, was related to the increase of pre-adolescents' adherence. However, these authors [42] did not find any association between authoritative parenting and improved metabolic control as observed among this parenting style and adherence. One reason for this fact may be due to glycated hemoglobin being on average under 8.0%, i.e., pre-adolescents who participated in this study showed a metabolic control recommended by ADA [20], for this age group, that delay medical complications.

Additionally uninvolved family style was related to poor self-management and poor quality of life [43]. When neither the parent or the adolescents assume the responsibility for diabetes care, or adolescents have excessive autonomy in diabetes management, adolescents presented worse metabolic control [18, 35]. For that reason, even during adolescence, the family must continue involved in diabetes management tasks, and the responsibility for diabetes care should be gradually transferred to adolescent only when they demonstrate the maturity and the adequate capacities to lead with the diabetes management tasks [22].

Emotional support of parents and parental responsiveness were related with a better quality of life in adolescents with diabetes [3]. Also Jaser and Grey [36] emphasized the family influence on adolescents' quality of life, concluding that warmth and family caring behaviors were related to better quality of life in adolescents. That same study showed that observed intrusive parenting behaviors, like parental influence, were related to adolescents' quality of life and depressive symptoms. Furthermore, Pereira, Berg-Cross, Almeida and Machado [33] found that family conflicts were a predictor of less quality of life in adolescents with diabetes. Family conflict among T1DM adolescents and their parents were related to lower quality of life in adolescents [9] and were also associated with several psychological and behavioral outcomes in young adolescents with T1DM [34].

6. Conclusion

During adolescence, the balance between developmental struggles, challenges and family interactions represent a delicate and crucial component of a successful process of adaptation to diabetes that include an optimal metabolic control and a good quality of life, in T1DM adolescent.

Communication between parents and adolescents seems to have an important influence either on adolescent's adjustment to diabetes or in glycemic results or quality of life. Thus, interventions which allow the development of communication skills related to diabetes management in T1DM adolescents and their parents may decrease family conflicts and improve adolescent's metabolic control.

Interventions to develop self-management and decision-making in T1DM adolescents and their families also appear to be useful to improve adolescents' metabolic control and quality of life. It is important in order to improve adolescent outcomes, that adolescents develop their diabetes self-management skills and learn how to share diabetes responsibility with parents, without engaging in family conflicts.

Parents of T1DM adolescents must develop a collaborative parenting style with adolescents in their diabetes management and appropriated levels of guidance and control to improve adolescents' metabolic control and quality of life and, simultaneously, minimize family conflicts over diabetes management.

Author details

Ana Cristina Almeida[1], Engrácia Leandro[2] and Maria da Graça Pereira[3*]

*Address all correspondence to: gracep@psi.uminho.pt

1 University of Minho, Social Sciences Institute; Braga, Portugal

2 Researcher at Centre for Research and Studies in Sociology, University Institute of Lisbon; Lisbon, Portugal

3 University of Minho, School of Psychology; Braga, Portugal

References

[1] Jaser SS, Whittemore R, Ambrosino JM, Lindemann E, Grey M. Mediators of Depressive Symptoms in Children with Type 1 Diabetes and their Mothers. Journal of Pediatric Psychology. 2008;3(5):509-519. DOI: 10.1093/jpepsy/jsm104

[2] Cohen DM, Lumley MA, Naar-King S, Partridge T, Cakan N. Child Behavior Problems and Family Functioning as Predictors of Adherence and Glycemic Control in Economically Disadvantaged Children with Type 1 Diabetes: A Prospective Study. Journal of Pediatric Psychology. 2004;29(3):171-184. DOI: 10.1093/jpepsy/jsh019

[3] Moore SM, Hackworth NJ, Hamilton VE, Northam EP, Cameron FJ. Adolescents with Type 1 Diabetes: Parental Perceptions of Child Health and Family Functioning and Their Relationship to Adolescent Metabolic Control. Health and Quality of Life Outcomes. 2013;11(50):8. DOI: 10.1186/1477-7525-11-50

[4] Whittemore R. Strategies to Facilitate Lifestyle Change Associated with Diabetes Mellitus. Journal of Nursing Scholarship. 2000;32(3):225-232. DOI: 10.1111/j.1547-5069.2000.00225.x

[5] Chao A, Whittemore R, Minges KE, Murphy KM, Grey M. Self-Management in Early Adolescence and Differences by Age at Diagnosis and Duration of Type 1 Diabetes. The Diabetes Educator. 2014;40(2):167-177. DOI: 10.1177/0145721713520567

[6] Whittemore R, Jaser S, Chao A, Jang M, Grey M. Psychological Experience of Parents of Children With Type 1 Diabetes: A Systematic Mixed-Studies Review. The Diabetes Educator. 2012;38(4):562-579. DOI: 10.1177/0145721712445216

[7] Guo J, Whittemore R, He G-P. The Relationship between Diabetes Self-Management and Metabolic Control in Youth with Type 1 Diabetes: An Integrative Review. Journal of Advanced Nursing. 2011;67(11):2294-2310. DOI: 10.1111/j.1365-2648.2011.05697.x

[8] La Greca AM, Thompson KM. Family and Friend Support for Adolescents with Diabetes. Análise Psicológica. 1998;16(1):101-113.

[9] De Wit M, De Waal HA, Bokma JA, Haasnoot K, Houdijk MC, Gemke RJ, *et al.* Self-Report and Parent-Report of Physical and Psychosocial Well-Being in Dutch Adoles-

cents with Type 1 Diabetes in Relation to Glycemic Control. Health and Quality of Life Outcomes. 2007;5(10). DOI: 10.1186/1477-7525-5-10

[10] Malik JA, Koot HM. Explaining the Adjustment of Adolescents with Type 1 Diabetes. Role of Diabetes-Specific and Psychosocial Factors. Diabetes Care. 2009;32:774-779. DOI: 10.2337/dc08-1306

[11] Grey M, Whittemore R, Jeon S, Murphy K, Faulkner MS, Delamater A. Internet Psycho-Education Programs Improve Outcomes in Youth with Type 1 Diabetes. Diabetes Care. 2013;36:2475-2482. DOI: 10.2337/dc12-2199

[12] Jaser SS, Faulkner MS, Whittemore R, Jeon S, Murphy K, Delamater A, *et al.* Coping, Self-Management, and Adaptation in Adolescents with Type 1 Diabetes. Annals of Behavioral Medicine. 2012;43:311-319. DOI: 10.1007/s12160-012-9343-z

[13] Kalyva E, Malakonaki E, Eiser C, Mamoulakis D. Health-Related Quality of Life (HRQoL) of Children with Type 1 Diabetes Mellitus (T1DM): Self and Parental Perceptions. Pediatric Diabetes. 2011;12:34-40. DOI: 10.1111/j.1399-5448.2010.00653.x

[14] Jaser SS. Psychological Problems in Adolescents with Diabetes. Adolescent Medicine: State of the Art Reviews. 2010;21(1):138-151.

[15] Whittemore R, Jaser S, Guo J, Grey M. A Conceptual Model of Childhood Adaptation to Type 1 Diabetes. Nursing Outlook. 2010;58:242-251. DOI: 10.1016/j.outlook.2010.05.001

[16] Butner J, Berg CA, Osborn P, Butler JM, Godri C, Fortenberry KT *et al.* Parent-Adolescent Discrepancies in Adolescents' Competence and the Balance of Adolescent Autonomy and Adolescent and Parent Well-Being in the Context of Type 1 Diabetes. Developmental Psychology. 2009;45(3):835-849. DOI: 10.1037/a0015363

[17] Guo J, Whittemore R, Jeon S, Grey M, Zhou Z-G, He G-P *et al.* Diabetes Self-Management, Depressive Symptoms, Metabolic Control and Satisfaction with Quality of Life over Time in Chinese Youth with Type 1 Diabetes. Journal of Clinical Nursing. 2014;26. DOI: 10.1111/jocn.12698

[18] Faulkner MS, Chang L-I. Family Influence on Self-Care, Quality of Life, and Metabolic Control in School-Age Children and Adolescents with Type 1 Diabetes. Journal of Pediatric Nursing. 2007;22(1):59-68. DOI: 10.1016/j.pedn.2006.02.008

[19] Kyngäs H. Compliance of Adolescents with Chronic Disease. Journal of Clinical Nursing. 2000;9(4):549-556. DOI: 10.1046/j.1365-2702.2000.00368.x

[20] American Diabetes Association (ADA). Standards of Medical Care in Diabetes – 2010. Diabetes Care. 2010;33(1):S11-S61. DOI: 10.2337/dc10-S011

[21] Hoey H. Psychosocial Factors are Associated with Metabolic Control in Adolescents: Research from the Hvidoere Study Group on Childhood Diabetes. Pediatric Diabetes. 2009;10(13):9-14. DOI: 10.1111/j.1399-5448.2009.00609.x

[22] Malerbi FE, Negrato CA, Gomes MB. Assessment of Psychosocial Variables by Parents of Youth with Type 1 Diabetes Mellitus. Diabetology & Metabolic Syndrome. 2012;4(48). DOI: 10.1186/1758-5996-4-48

[23] Wysocki T, Greco P. Social Support and Diabetes Management in Childhood and Adolescence: Influence of Parents and Friends. Current Diabetes Reports. 2006;6(2): 117-122. DOI: 10.1007/s11892-006-0022-y

[24] Lewin AB, Heidgerken AD, Geffken GR, Williams LB, Storch EA, Gelfand KM. The Relation Between Family Factors and Metabolic Control: The Role of Diabetes Adherence. Journal of Pediatric Psychology. 2006;31(2):174-183. DOI: 10.1093/jpepsy/jsj004

[25] Grey M, Jaser SS, Whittemore R, Jeon S, Lindemann E. Coping Skills Training for Parents of Children with Type 1 Diabetes: 12-Month Outcomes. Nursing Research and Practice. 2011;60(3):173-181. DOI: 10.1097/NNR.0b013e3182159c8f

[26] Al-Akor N, Khader YS, Shatnawi NJ. Quality of Life and Associated Factors Among Jordanian Adolescents with Type 1 Diabetes Mellitus. Journal of Diabetes and Its Complications. 2010;24(1):43-47. DOI: 10.1016/j.jdiacomp.2008.12.011

[27] Pereira M, Almeida A, Rocha L, Leandro E. Predictors of Adherence, Metabolic Control and Quality of Life in Adolescents with Type 1 Diabetes. In: Liu C-P, editor. Type 1 Diabetes – Complications, Pathogenesis, and Alternative Treatments. Rijeka: InTech; 2011. p. 119-140. DOI: 10.5772/24042

[28] Guttmann-Bauman I, Flaherty BP, Strugger M, McEvoy RC. Metabolic Control and Quality-of-Life Self-Assessment in Adolescents with IDDM. Diabetes Care. 1998;21(6):915-918. DOI: 10.2337/diacare.21.6.915

[29] Glasgow RE, Ruggiero L, Eakin EG, Dryfoos J, Chobanian L. Quality of Life and Associated Characteristics in a Large National Sample of Adults with Diabetes. Diabetes Care. 1997;20(4):532-567. DOI: 10.2337/diacare.20.4.562

[30] Fogel NR, Weissberg-Benchell J. Preventing Poor Psychological and Health Outcomes in Pediatric Type 1 Diabetes. Current Diabetes Reports. 2010;10(6):436-443. DOI: 10.1007/s11892-010-0145-z

[31] Matziou V, Tsoumakas K, Vlahioti E, Chrysicopoulou L, Galanis P, Petsios K et al. Factors Influencing the Quality of Life of Young Patients with Diabetes. Journal of Diabetes. 2011;3(1):82-90. DOI: 10.1111/j.1753-0407.2010.00106.x

[32] Guo J, Whittemore R, Grey M, Wang J, Zhou Z-G, He G-P. Diabetes Self-Management, Depressive Symptoms, Quality of Life and Metabolic Control in Youth with Type 1 Diabetes in China. Journal of Clinical Nursing. 2012;22(1-2):69-79. DOI: 10.1111/j.1365-2702.2012.04299.x

[33] Pereira MG, Berg-Cross L, Almeida P, Machado CJ. Impact of Family Environment and Support on Adherence, Metabolic Control, and Quality of Life in Adolescents

with Diabetes. International Journal of Behavioral Medicine. 2008;15:187-193. DOI: 10.1080/10705500802222436

[34] Whittemore R, Liberti L, Jeon S, Chao A, Jaser SS, Grey M. Self-Management as a Mediator of Family Functioning and Depressive Symptoms with Health Outcomes in Youth with Type 1 Diabetes. Western Journal of Nursing Research. 2014;36(9): 1254-1271. DOI: 10.1177/0193945913516546

[35] Skinner TC, John M, Hampson SE. Social Support and Personal Models of Diabetes as Predictors of Self-Care and Well-Being: A Longitudinal Study of Adolescents with Diabetes. Journal of Pediatric Psychology. 2000;25(4):257-267. DOI: 10.1093/jpepsy/25.4.257

[36] Jaser SS, Grey M. A Pilot Study of Observed Parenting and Adjustment in Adolescents with Type 1 Diabetes and their Mothers. Journal of Pediatric Psychology. 2010;35(7):738-747. DOI: 10.1093/jpepsy/jsp098

[37] Duke DC, Geffken GR, Lewin AB, Williams LB, Storch EA, Silverstein JH. Glycemic Control in Youth with Type 1 Diabetes: Family Predictors and Mediators. Journal of Pediatric Psychology. 2008;33(7):719-727. DOI: 10.1093/jpepsy/jsn012

[38] McKelvey J, Waller DA, North, AJ, Marks JF, Schreiner B, Travis LB, Murphy JN. Reliability and Validity of the Diabetes Family Behavior Scale (DFBS). The Diabetes Educator. 1993;19(2):125-132.

[39] Wysocki T, Linschied TR, Taylor A, Yeates KO, Hough BS, Naglieri JA. Deviation from Developmentally Appropriate Self-Care Autonomy. Diabetes Care. 1996;19(2): 119-125. DOI: 10.2337/diacare.19.2.119

[40] Tsiouli E, Alexapoulos EC, Stefanaki C, Darviri C, Chrousos GP. Effects of Diabetes-Related Family Stress on Glycemic Control in Young Patients with Type 1 Diabetes. Canadian Family Physician. 2013;59(2):143-149.

[41] Anderson BJ. Family Conflict and Diabetes Management in Youth: Clinical Lessons from Child Development and Diabetes Research. Diabetes Spectrum. 2004;17(1): 22-26. DOI: 10.2337/diaspect.17.1.22

[42] Monaghan M, Horn IV, Alvarez V, Cogen FR, Streisand R. Authoritative Parenting, Parenting Stress, and Self-Care in Pre-Adolescents with Type 1 Diabetes. Journal of Clinical Psychology in Medical Settings. 2012;19(3):255-261. DOI: 10.1007/s10880-011-9284-x

[43] Laffel L, Connell A, Vangsness L, Goebel-Fabri A, Mansfield A, Anderson B. General Quality of Life in Youth with Type 1 Diabetes. Relationship to Patient Management and Diabetes-Specific Family Conflict. Diabetes Care. 2003;26(11):3067-3073. DOI: 10.2337/diacare.26.11.3067

Chapter 8

Improving Adherence for Children with Diabetes

Laura Nabors, Teminijesu John Ige, Alicia Aikens, Chris Berry,
Bradley Fevrier and Patrice DeLeon

Additional information is available at the end of the chapter

http://dx.doi.org/10.5772/60567

Abstract

This chapter provides critical information on diabetes in children. Ideas for improving adherence to the child's medical regimen are reviewed. In addition, factors that may hinder adherence are presented. Ideas for clinicians are presented in a case study.

Keywords: Children, diabetes, adherence

1. Introduction

Within the last two decades, diabetes mellitus (DM) has been reported with increased frequency among children and adolescents in the United States and has become one of the more common chronic illnesses among this population (Centers for Disease Control and Prevention (CDC) [1]). According to the CDC's SEARCH for Diabetes among Youth Study, over 200, 000 people younger than 20 years have DM, with type 1 diabetes (T1DM) being more prevalent (1.93 for every 1, 000 young people), except among American Indian youth where it is less prevalent than type 2 diabetes (T2DM) [1, 2]. The prevalence rate of T2DM in the general population of youth is much less (0.24 per 1, 000 young people [1, 2]. With regard to incidence, an estimated 28.1 cases of DM occur per 100, 000 youth per year—18, 436 youth (about 19.7 per 100, 000) are diagnosed with T1DM, and 5, 089 (about 8.5 per 100, 000) are diagnosed with T2DM [1]. Within the past 20 years, the incidence of T2DM has increased, which may be attributable to the concurrent epidemic of overweight and obesity [3]. T1DM is most common among white youth followed by Hispanic and African American youth. T2DM more commonly occurs among American Indian and African American youth and is least common among Asian/Pacific Islander and non-Hispanic white youth. Asian/Pacific Islander youth have, on average, the least incidence and prevalence of both types of diabetes [1, 2].

The health issues faced by adolescent diabetics are similar to those experienced by adults, especially as they mature into adulthood (National Diabetes Education Program, NDEP) [4]. These issues include maintaining optimal blood glucose (glycemic) control, weight management, healthy nutrition, proper physical exercise, and prevention of long-term complications such as diabetic eye disease, diabetic renal disease, diabetic vascular disease, and diabetic nerve disease. Poor glycemic control manifests acutely as hypoglycemia and diabetic ketoacidosis, and chronically as health complications such as retinopathy and nerve damage [3, 4]. Both acute manifestations of poor glycemic control are potentially fatal and more so in youth who may not be fully cognizant of the symptoms, especially while at play. It is therefore important for diabetic youth and those who care for them to be properly educated about the symptoms, signs, and management of these conditions, and to be trained on maintaining optimal blood glucose control, which also helps to delay the onset of complications [3, 4].

Overweight and obesity have become increasingly important health issues in young diabetics. This is due to the rapid rise in cases of T2DM among this population within the last 20 years. T2DM in youth has been found to be associated with overweight and obesity, and therefore weight control has become an important component in the management of the disease [3, 5]. Nutrition is also a major issue in diabetic youth because healthful nutrition helps with blood glucose control, weight management, and maintenance of an optimum nutritional status necessary to maintain good health, boost immunity, and help prevent complications [4, 6]. Physical exercise is another important health issue. Diabetics tend to avoid physical exercise due to fear of hypoglycemia and other short-term effects of physical stress [4]. However, while blood glucose control is a concern during exercise, physical exercise has been shown to improve the health and quality of life of diabetics especially since it helps with weight and blood glucose control, improves blood circulation, and increases insulin sensitivity, thus reducing the complications associated with the disease [3, 4, 7]. It is important to encourage exercise in diabetic youth, create exercise regimens that meet their needs, and ensure proper supervision by experienced fitness instructors trained in diabetic exercise management and blood glucose control [4].

2. Problem

In the remainder of this chapter, we address adherence for children and adolescents with diabetes. The majority of our information will address issues for youth with T1DM, although more research on adherence for youth with T2DM is needed.

3. Defining adherence

Adherence is a focal point of this chapter, and in subsequent sections of this chapter, we discuss other factors related to adherence, successful interventions, and ideas for improving child adherence. The World Health Organization (WHO) has developed an inclusive definition of adherence, which we believe encompasses health care needs of youth with diabetes as well as other types of chronic illnesses [8]. The WHO, in a report on long-term therapies for those with chronic illnesses edited by Sabate, described adherence (and we paraphrase their ideas) as behaviors indicating an individual was following medical and lifestyle recommendations related to a chronic illness [8]. Adherence is thus important to maintaining health and a good quality of life when a child or individual is facing a chronic condition. In the following section of this chapter, we discuss key items for adherence for children with diabetes, focusing chiefly on the importance of diet and exercise as long-term contributors to a healthy lifestyle.

In a recent study examining adherence to clinical practice guidelines, Amed et al. [9] reported that only about 7–8% of youth with T1DM were meeting national and international adherence practice guidelines. Moreover, they also indicated that children and adolescents who had been struggling with their diabetes for a longer period of time (i.e., had a longer time since diagnosis [4+ years]) were apt to have poor adherence and caretaking of their diabetes. Adherence is also a problem for youth with T2DM, and more youth are coping with T2DM and facing the same types of negative health outcomes as faced by children and adolescents with T1DM and as adults with T2DM [10]. Obese youth may be at a very high risk for T2DM, and increasing intake of fruits and vegetables and decreasing intake of foods high in fat and sugar may reduce health risks for these youth.

4. Factors related to adherence and health

4.1. Health risks

Youth with either T1DM or T2DM (usually older children) may face significant health risks. Microvascular risks, which can be lessened when glycemic control remains good, include nephropathy, retinopathy, and neuropathy. Similar to adults, children may face macrovascular risks (e.g., cardiovascular problems) as a long-term complication related to their diabetes [11]. Macrovascular risks also may be attenuated with good glycemic control, making adherence a key health topic for children and adolescents as the patterns and behaviors they establish as youth will impact their health quality in later years. Youth with T2DM may also face significant health challenges related to obesity, making cardiovascular health particularly important. One study assessing outcomes for youth with T2DM may provide a wealth of information for those interested in learning about health outcomes for youth with T2DM. This study is entitled the Treatment Options for Type 2 Diabetes in Adolescents and Youth (TODAY) study, and this is a well-designed multisite study funded by the National Institute of Diabetes and Digestive Kidney Diseases [10].

4.2. Isolation

Social isolation can be a negative experience for individuals with diabetes. Marrero et al. [12] proposed that peer support can reduce isolation and provide support for the diabetes patient in reaching his or her goals. Support from health professionals and clinicians also can be critical to reducing isolation. Support can also be provided "online." For example, Nicholas et al. [13] reported that adolescents with diabetes who received online support were less likely to feel isolated because they had diabetes. Adolescents in the online program showed enhanced knowledge about their diabetes. Results from qualitative interviews indicated that adolescents reported reduced feelings of isolation, and they felt less "different" after participating in online support and education groups. Some adolescents in an 8-week online educational and support group reported improved quality of support from others outside their family; however, these results were not robust, and further research on the "support" gained from online groups is needed.

4.3. Problems with emotional functioning

Older children and adolescents experiencing stress may have poorer immune system functioning and have poorer glycemic control [14]. Thus, the experience of stress may exacerbate problems with diabetes management, making adherence an important tool in combating the stress-poor glycemic control link. In addition, females and youth in ethnic minority groups may report higher levels of stress, indicating a greater need for support in helping them maintain optimal glucose levels. Delamater et al. reported that youth (participants in their study were aged 9–20 years) were clearly stressed over their diet. Health professionals need to assess adolescent stress levels and converse with adolescents to determine when referral for counseling to problem-solve coping with stressors and develop plans for improving adherence is needed. Working with children and adolescents to develop a strong relationship to be able to assess child functioning and have rapport so that the youngster remains positive about referral for supportive counseling is important as well to ensure that referrals themselves are considered positive by the youth. Stress also may be related to poor glycemic control for youth with T2DM. For example, Walders-Abramson and colleagues [15] from the Treatment Options for Type 2 Diabetes in Adolescents and Youth Study Group found that for youth with T2DM the odds of having difficulty with adherence to their medication regimen increased if they were experiencing difficulty with significant life stressors. They also found increased depression among youth coping with significant stressors, and this variable may also impact adherence for youth with T2DM [15].

Similarly, suffering from symptoms related to depression, a common problem for youth with T1DM, may be related to poor adherence to diabetic regimens [16]. In a meta-analysis and systematic review of the literature, Kongkaew et al. [17] found a relationship between feelings of depression and problems with adherence in youth with diabetes. They recommended working with adolescents to improve adherence behaviors in addition to working with adolescents to improve their mood [17]. Working on improving mood may indirectly improve adherence because if one feels happier, it may be easier to manage diabetes self-care. Researchers have reported that other variables, in addition to depressed mood, may interact to influence adherence problems, including appetite disturbance, poor self-care skills, or experiencing significant life stressors [15, 16]. Thus, additional studies assessing self-care, stressful life events, and emotional stressors are needed to begin to understand the pathways to poor adherence in adolescents experiencing emotional distress.

Herzer and Hood reported that adolescents with diabetes may experience relatively high levels of anxiety [18]. These researchers found that higher state anxiety (e.g., anxiety related to daily stressors) was related to less frequent monitoring of blood glucose levels and poorer glycemic control. Although anxiety may be less prominent than depression and less common in younger children, they too may experience anxiety related to their diabetes management [19]. Hence, it remains essential for clinicians and health professionals to monitor children's feelings of

http://dx.doi.org/10.5772/60567

worry and concern over their diabetes management and health risks related to this chronic illness. Health professionals can assist children and adolescents in identifying the aforementioned feelings and educating children about how tension and worry can negatively impact their motivation to follow their diabetes regimen. It is important to point out that being anxious and not following the regimen can actually lead to more feelings of anxiety as blood glucose levels remain too high as a consequence of poor adherence to dietary guidelines, insulin administration, etc. Buckloh et al. [11] conducted focus groups with parents and caregivers for youth with T1DM and found that parents also were experiencing anxiety related to adherence issues with their child as well as evolving anxiety related to possible long-term complications related to their child's diabetes. Hence, focusing on anxiety in parents and children and how to reduce anxiety related to adhering to diet, exercise, testing blood glucose levels, and insulin administration will assist the entire family's coping, which may have a positive impact on glucose monitoring and glycemic control. Improving exercise and teaching parents and children relaxation skills (e.g., breathing and positive imagery) may be helpful anxiety management strategies.

In this section on emotional functioning, we have focused primarily on internalizing symptoms, namely, depression and anxiety, in youth with T1DM. It is noteworthy that youth with T1DM can experience a myriad of psychological problems, related to both internalizing (e.g., anxiety and depression) and externalizing (i.e., acting out) symptoms related to conduct problems [19]. It will remain important to continue to examine the relations among conduct problems and other mental health issues such as attention problems and oppositional behaviors to improve our understanding of how emotional problems impact adherence. Furthermore, there is relatively less literature on emotional problems and adherence for adolescents with T2DM, and this will be another area for future study.

5. Application areas

Youth with T1DM work to adhere to insulin administration, typically using the diabetes pump. They also must count their carbohydrates in order to regulate intake of carbohydrates. They must juggle monitoring blood glucose levels and administering insulin as well as managing their stress, diet, and exercise, which all can have a significant impact on their diabetes management.

Youth with T2DM struggle with adherence to taking medications regularly. In a recent study, the Today Study Group or Today Group reported that administration of two medications—metformin and rosiglitazone—improved diabetes management, especially for girls [10]. Youth do struggle with taking medications regularly, and like their counterparts with T1DM, those with T2DM also must work to monitor their diet, exercise, and stress levels. Interestingly, the lifestyle intervention employed in the study by the Today Group did not provide "value added" to glycemic control over and above the medications. The Today Group concluded that more fine-grained analysis of the lifestyle intervention and further study of interventions to improve adherence among youth this T2DM will be needed [10]. In the next paragraphs of this section on key areas for adherence, we will review research conducted with youth with T1DM as the majority of research is with children with T1DM. However, more research on dietary and exercise adherence for youth with T2DM will advance knowledge about optimal care for youth with T2DM.

After conducting a multisite study in Brazil, Davison and colleagues [20] in the Brazilian Type 1 Diabetes Study Group indicated that approximately 54% of the youth with T1DM in their sample were adherent to their diet, which these researchers defined as following the diet about 80% of the time. There were over 3, 000 patients in the sample for this study and these youth had participated in medical follow-up for at least 1 year. Surprisingly, only about 12% were following a diet prescribed by the Brazilian Diabetes Society, and 48% of the patients followed a diet of avoiding sweets and sugar. Moreover, it was unclear about whether they were knowledgeable about the importance of counting carbohydrates to maintain good glycemic control. Problems with glycemic control were evident in this sample. Adherence to dietary guidelines was associated with lower rates of hyperglycemia and ketoacidosis, but adherence to the diet was not associated with episodes of hypoglycemia [20].

Adherence to dietary guidelines for children and adolescents with type 1diabetes involves a balance of carbohydrate and insulin levels to maintain recommended blood glucose levels. In a review of studies examining nutrition of children with T1DM, Patton [21] discovered that youth with diabetes may consume more fruits and vegetables than their peers. We believe that after investigating the eating habits of clients with diabetes, health professionals should praise the eating habits of youth with diabetes if they are making efforts to consume more fruits and vegetables. On the other hand, Patton also mentioned that these youth may need to watch and also reduce their fat consumption [21]. In addition to teaching youth to count carbohydrates, paying attention to the general health level of the youth's diet may contribute to helping them engage in healthy habits. We recommend that children become involved in learning about healthy eating and that health professionals and parents use rewards and encouragement to assist children in setting and achieving dietary goals. For very young children, using games and immediate rewards for trying new healthy foods may be a good way to involve them in plans for healthy eating.

Patton et al. [22] found that adherence to insulin administration is one cornerstone of good management, and in addition, eating a healthy diet and managing carbohydrate intake further helps manage diabetes. Self-monitoring charts, to track insulin administration, may help youth and their parents follow recommendations for regular testing of blood glucose levels. Incentives can be used to encourage youth to improve the regularity with which they test blood glucose levels. Some youngsters may be more likely to remember to test with reminders from an adult, and then the boy or girl can work toward more independent blood glucose monitoring and more control over self-monitoring schedules.

Our team wanted to highlight the importance of increasing knowledge about the impact of physical activity for children. Engaging in regular physical activity may be a key ingredient for glycemic control for youth with diabetes. Quirk et al. [23] reviewed studies from 1964 to 2012 on the effectiveness of physical activity for children and adolescents with diabetes (youth were between 8 and 17 years of age). They discovered 26 studies, and in 23 of these studies, there was at least one positive outcome for children and adolescents who engaged in exercise.

However, in the studies reviewed, the length of the physical activity interventions varied between 2 and 39 weeks. The type of exercise also varied; some studies assessed engagement in one exercise (e.g., walking, swimming), and in other studies, several types of activities were used (e.g., cycling, games with balls, lifting weights, circuit training). Thus, there was great variety in the studies under review. Quirk et al. did find that engaging in physical activity had a moderate impact on glycosated hemoglobin levels, which is positive. Studies were often atheoretical and did not address change in motivation or psychological variables [23]. Future research on the impact of physical activity and the psychological variables associated with engagement in regular physical activity will advance knowledge about how activity affects children and adolescents with diabetes.

6. Research on factors related to adherence

6.1. Family relationships and communication

The support that the child receives from his or her family can positively impact diabetes management, and this includes adherence to medical regimens. Positive support occurs when the family allows for individuality and has open communication about medical management. Open communication allows the child to provide input and involves respecting his or her personality. We recommend regular family meetings to discuss how the family is coping and to discuss diabetes management so that a pattern of open communication can develop. Rules in the family should be consistently applied and remain flexible [24]. Within the family, the parent–child relationship can be the key factor determining positive steps toward adhering to the medical regimen. This relationship and the communication during mealtimes and snack times also can influence adherence [22].

Family support for diabetes management (especially for tasks needed to manage the illness on a daily basis) is related to improved adherence and ultimately improved metabolic control [25]. It is important for parents to remain flexible at mealtimes and in their communications with their child and to not appear too critical in order to engage the child and promote positive conversations about measuring carbohydrate intake and ensuring a healthy diet. Having open communication can help the child and parent by opening opportunities to discuss the child's goals and areas for improving monitoring of diabetes management. Adolescent disclosure is essential to high parental knowledge and positive adolescent adjustments to diabetes adherence. On the other hand, nondisclosure and secrecy on the part of the adolescent has been shown to be related to greater symptoms of depression among adolescents trying to manage their diabetes [26]. Some adolescents may be likely to keep secrets about those times they "slip" in terms of adhering to their diabetes care; therefore, parents may want to ask adolescents about slips and promote an atmosphere of correcting, but not admonishing slips, so that adolescents can talk to them about snacking and appropriate corrections to insulin dosages can be made. Disclosure on the part of adolescents may be more important for mothers compared to fathers [26]; however, this is an area for further study.

6.2. Youth involvement in decision making

Developing specific daily and weekly goals for diabetes management may be another protective factor to ensure that children and adolescents remain "on track" in terms of following their diabetes regimen. Youth should be involved in setting goals and providing input on plans to improve their adherence. In fact, joint decision making between parents and youth with diabetes may be one way to improve youth involvement in their diabetes care [27]. Involving them in decisions may improve their adherence to their diet and other aspects of their medical regimen. Miller and Jawad encouraged caregivers and other health care professionals to inspire youth with diabetes to express their views [27]. We believe that this is important, and we also recommend that longitudinal, qualitative research be conducted to examine what type of shared management and decision making should occur for youth of different ages residing in various family situations.

6.3. School and after-school activities

A literature search for this chapter revealed that there is relatively less information available discussing children's ideas about what children and adolescents need to facilitate their diabetes management at school. This is unfortunate, given that children and adolescents typically view management at school as a significant issue. Nabors et al. [28] assessed children's perceptions of supports needed for their diabetes management at school. Children mentioned that support for individual care plans is needed. Some reported that they needed more snacks available or support from a peer in walking to see the nurse. Some children also wanted to check their blood glucose outside of the classroom in order to have some privacy [28]. The American Diabetes Association has developed guidelines for care of children with diabetes at school [29]. We recommend that health professionals or the medical team working with school-based management review these guidelines and then plan to meet with children, their parents or caregivers, and the school nurse to individualize care plans for the children, which are then shared with teachers. Very little information is available about the support that children need for participation in after-school and extracurricular activities, and this is an area for additional research.

6.4. Peer support

In a review of qualitative studies (from 2005 to 2011) of youth with diabetes, Ritholz et al. [30] discussed difficulties with interpersonal relationships as being a burden to some patients with diabetes. When reviewing studies focusing on children, they found that parents and family were sometimes perceived as supportive but could hinder an adolescent's or child's ability to socialize when not supporting their independence in attending social events. Parents also reported concerns about their child's growing independence in the adolescent years when he or she would have to manage his or her diabetes more independently in social situations [30]. Parents can become anxious about their child's ability to manage his or her diabetes regimen in social situations involving food or those where a child would be noticed as doing something different if he or she had to test his or her blood glucose level or administer insulin. Dr. Nabors, an author for this chapter, has worked with children at diabetes camps for several years. In

http://dx.doi.org/10.5772/60567

groups at camp, children have reported that attending camp is very beneficial for reducing feelings of isolation and feelings of being "the only one who is different." Involving children and adolescents with diabetes in peer support networks, with other same-aged youth with diabetes, may be an important way to reduce feelings of isolation for children and adolescents with diabetes. Marrero et al. supported the notion of peer support to reduce isolation and provide support for the diabetes patient in reaching his or her goals [12]. Support from health professionals and clinicians also can be critical to reducing isolation and sharing ideas that will both encourage and educate children with diabetes.

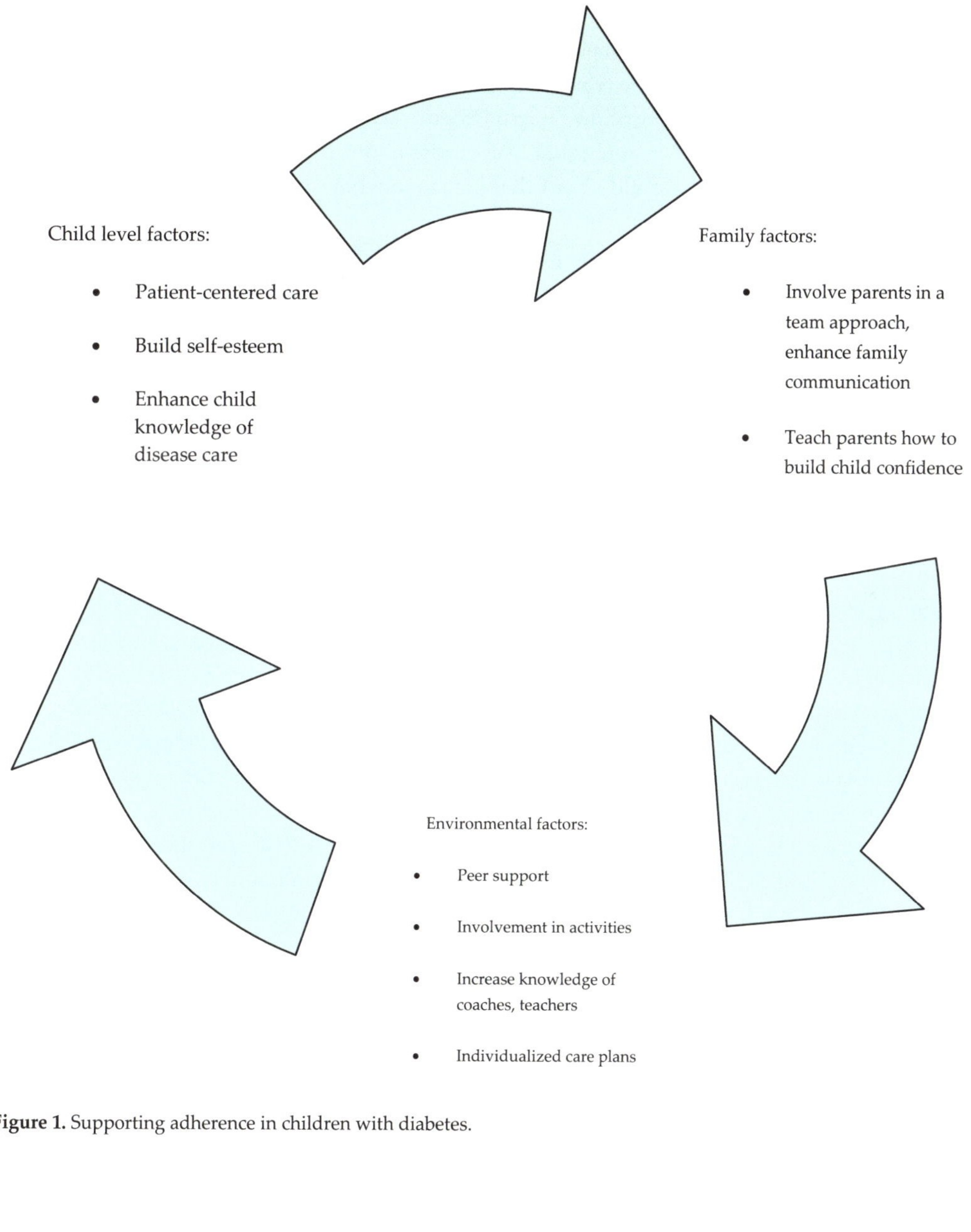

Figure 1. Supporting adherence in children with diabetes.

Figure 1 presents ideas for supporting a child as he or she copes with diabetes and the challenges of adhering to his or her medical regimen. It is important to consider that these factors interact and reciprocally influence each other. We believe that this graphic may assist health professionals in designing support plans for youth that focus on child, family, and environmental factors that will enhance support for following the medical regimen.

7. Adherence

7.1. Interventions to improve adherence

In a recent meta-analysis of 21 studies, Hood and colleagues [31] found a strong relationship between adherence and metabolic control in children and adolescents with T1DM. One key component of successful interventions is psychoeducation, aimed at educating parents of children with diabetes [32]. When parents learn more about diabetes management, they can better care for and teach their child about diabetes management tasks. When parents realize the importance of following the medical regimen, they are more likely to closely monitor and follow guidelines for diet, exercise, and glucose monitoring provided by their child's medical team. We believe that parent education and ongoing support from the medical team, to maintain education with booster sessions to adapt parent training to the child's age, self-efficacy for diabetes management, and family routines, are important. The child's medical team can provide booster sessions to enhance parent knowledge and provide needed support to parents on an as-needed basis. Online interventions to educate parents may also be effective in educating them and linking them to support from the medical team and other parents, as in the Dutch Sugarsquare intervention [33]. Internet education may be especially important in rural areas or when parents lack transportation to access care in hospital settings to participate in support groups.

Health professionals can improve adherence. Patient-centered care will be important in developing plans that work for individual children and their family members. Kienle et al. [34, p. 13] stated, "The cornerstone of diabetic care is comprehensive case management including intense education to enable self-management adjusted for the child's age and developmental stage and with assistance from caring and knowledgeable adults." In their manuscript, Kienle et al. reported on a case study to improve child involvement in diabetes management for a girl with diabetes and other special needs. A patient-centered approach with repeated educational sessions was used to improve the girls' involvement in her care. The aforementioned authors wrote that reeducation was critical to helping the girl as she learned and strove to improve her diabetes management. In the long run, the authors reported higher self-esteem and greater involvement in social activities [34]. Although children who do not have special needs may not need extensive reeducation, we believe that they can benefit from booster sessions or support groups, which allow review of the importance of adherence to dietary and exercise recommendations as well as reinforcing the importance of glucose monitoring.

We also believe that goal setting will be important for children and their parents. While setting goals, the child and parents should be involved in goal setting. As the child ages, parents can become less involved in leading goal-setting efforts. However, we believe that they should remain interested, caring, and involved on some level to support their adolescent. Evaluating alternatives to reach a level of good diabetes management, setting a plan, and breaking steps of the plan down into obtainable goals are part of an effective decision making process. After executing goals, it becomes important for the child/adolescent and family to evaluate the effectiveness of their plan, in terms of diabetes management and quality of life for the youth. Enhanced levels of positive communication from parents and lower negative communications from both parents and adolescents can improve communication, leading to better adherence [35]. Similarly, problem-solving skills may be another tool to teach children with diabetes to review situations in their lives and brainstorm about adherence issues and develop goals that will best assist them, within the context where they are, in managing their diabetes. Teaching children to advocate for themselves and what they need to manage their diabetes is another tool in helping them to be able to implement goals they have for themselves [36].

Marrero et al. [12] recommend that when assisting with goal setting, it is important that the individual feels that he or she can achieve them. They recommend key components of motivational interviewing as being consistent with a patient-centered model to promote self-management as the provider is developing attainable goals from the patient's own frame of reference and using encouragement and praise to help motivate the patient to achieve his or her goals. We believe that this patient-centered stance, to the extent possible with a child and parent or caregiver in a "shared" management approach, will foster self-efficacy for diabetes management and enhanced involvement in diabetes care for children as well as adolescents. We recommend setting goals related to carbohydrate counting and teaching children and adolescents about counting carbohydrates. A relatively recent study has shown this is an effective dietary technique with adults [37]. If carbohydrate counting begins in childhood, perhaps this method can become a more routine behavior in adolescence, making it relatively easier to allow the adolescent to have primary control in counting carbohydrates and dietary management.

After receiving education about diabetes management, text messaging and reminders may be a way to boost adherence. This may be because children, adolescents, and parents or caregivers may respond well to reminders to help them with monitoring adherence to diabetes regimens. It may be feasible for children to send information on their monitoring efforts via mobile phone to research staff. This method may result in successful support, and messaging may be a good method for providing booster sessions, in terms of reminders and short educational messages to improve adherence.

8. Case studies

The next paragraphs of this chapter present information related to adherence through case studies with fictional characters to review key issues related to adherence. This will illustrate key points in the research on adherence at an individual level.

8.1. Case study 1

Jacklyn is an 11-year-old white girl with T1DM. She has had diabetes since she turned 4 years old. She is the youngest of four children. She gets along well with her siblings and parents most of the time. She has one good friend at school and two close friends in her neighborhood. She enjoys dancing and belongs to a local dance group. Her grades at school remain strong, with a long-standing academic record of A's and B's.

Jacklyn has recently experienced stress because her older sister, whom she used to be very close to, is now spending the majority of her time with a new boyfriend. Also, her mother just began working full time. Previously, she had a part-time job at a local school. This meant her mother's schedule matched Jacklyn's schedule and therefore her mother was readily available to help her manage her diabetes regimen. She packed Jacklyn's lunch and cooked all of her meals and was home to help Jacklyn with snacking. Since her part-time job was at Jacklyn's school, her mother was always available to help Jacklyn if she had a hypoglycemic or hyperglycemic episode at school. She had snacks on hand to bring to Jacklyn's classroom. Jacklyn wears a diabetic pump, which she likes better than shots.

Currently Jacklyn's mother has begun a full-time job in a local bank. Thus, for the first time, Jacklyn is having opportunities to manage her diabetes more independently. However, this has been proving a difficult task for Jacklyn. She keeps forgetting her snack to bring to school. She is having difficulty preparing her snacks at home and remembering to test her blood sugar and call her mother with the results. Jacklyn's mother is concerned for her daughter's diabetes management and mentioned this to the diabetes educator at one of Jacklyn's regular clinic visits. The diabetes educator had several recommendations to assist Jacklyn with her diabetes management.

First, the diabetes educator provided Jacklyn with a self-monitoring book, where she could record her blood sugar levels. She taught Jacklyn to set the alarm on her iPad so that she would have a "reminder" to remember to check her blood sugar regularly when she was home alone after school before her mother came home from work. She talked with Jacklyn about snacks she could have and then worked with Jacklyn and her mother to help them get snacks ready, in correct proportions, so that Jacklyn could easily get a snack, with knowledge of the carbohydrates in the snack, after testing her blood sugar when this was called for, based on results of blood glucose monitoring.

The diabetes educator recommended that Jacklyn and her mother have nightly checks to determine how her diabetes management had gone each day. At these "check-in" meetings, they could brainstorm about ways to improve diabetes management or it was an opportunity for Jacklyn's mother to praise her new-found independence if self-monitoring was leading to regular "testing" and better dietary monitoring/management.

Jacklyn responded well to the prospect of participating in meetings and was very excited to have positive support as she began to tackle having greater levels of responsibility in management of her diabetes regimen. However, she did ask that some meetings occur during brief telephone contacts as she had a very busy social life and was involved in after-school activities.

The diabetes educator did request that there be one in-person mother–daughter session to address communication about diabetes management between mother and daughter.

In this session, Jacklyn worked with her mother and the diabetes educator, in a private session, to rehearse ways to let other girls in her peer group know that she needed to count her carbohydrates and snack "thoughtfully" in order to best manage her diabetes. In their group session, the diabetes educator, Jacklyn, and her mother worked on improving their communication so that Jacklyn could tell her mother when she ate extra portions of high-carbohydrate foods and had "extra" snacks, so that when they talked on the telephone, her mother could offer the best guidance about insulin administration on her pump. Jacklyn's mother acknowledged that she could be very overprotective of her daughter and would try to use text messages rather than phone checks to briefly "check in" with her daughter. Her mother admitted she needed to place more trust in Jacklyn to manage her snacking and communicate with her mother about her own ideas about how best to manage her diet. At the end of this session, both mother and daughter agreed to a few more sessions to discuss communication and teamwork around diabetes management.

For the next few sessions, Jacklyn showed some resistance to sharing information with her mother because she was worried that her mother would become angry with her related to her "extra" snacking. Although her mother was not as receptive as she could have been, with further counseling sessions, she became more open to listening to her daughter and working with her daughter to develop a shared decision-making approach to setting goals and managing diet to help Jacklyn take a greater role in managing her diabetes. After a few more in-person sessions, the diabetes educator moved to telephone contacts and text messages with Jacklyn to keep in contact and help her keep tracking her carbohydrates and remembering to test her blood sugar levels. In time, the need for telephone checks also was reduced, and Jacklyn contacted her diabetes educator for support when needed. Jacklyn and her mother maintained their weekly meetings so that they had a dedicated time to plan regarding meals, snacks, and weekly diabetes management goals.

Over time, Jacklyn made progress in becoming more involved in her diabetes management. She was more involved in counting her carbohydrates. She was more involved in decision making about what she ate and in managing her diabetes. Jacklyn and her mother worked with the diabetes educator to develop a plan for Jacklyn to improve her self-monitoring and record her blood sugar levels by developing a logging method by storing her numbers on her telephone in a "notes application." Jacklyn continued to exercise regularly, and her involvement in decisions about her diabetes management improved, which improved her belief in her ability to make good decisions about managing her diabetes and to have more of a role in managing her diabetes.

Jacklyn did not present with serious emotional issues related to her diabetes management. Should this have been the case, then referral to a child psychologist or mental health counselor may have been warranted. Addressing emotional issues, such as depression, can improve diabetes management [16, 17]. Jacklyn was experiencing some feelings of sadness related to spending less time with her sister. A possible other area to improve quality of life may have been to ensure that Jacklyn was involved in meaningful activities with friends. Ensuring that she had opportunities to socialize with peers may have further contributed to positive emotional functioning.

Jacklyn might have benefitted from participating in a diabetes support group or attending a summer camp with other youth with T1DM. She would then be able to access peer support. If she was feeling isolated and perhaps feeling that she was the "only child" who had diabetes, being with others could have alleviated loneliness. If she experienced feelings of isolation due to believing that her friends did not understand her medical condition, support from peers facing similar issues could have provided a boost to her spirits, thereby improving her self-efficacy for managing her illness.

Self-monitoring of eating behaviors and carbohydrate counts was very helpful in assisting this youngster in understanding what she needed to do in terms of next steps in her diabetes management. This is consistent with research indicating that self-monitoring of blood glucose levels is critical to diabetes management in youth with T1DM [38]. Developing monitoring plans, which can "fit in" with children's and adolescents' busy lifestyles, and which can help them communicate with their parents, can be a way to track progress and gather concrete data about ways to improve diabetes management. Calendars, tracking sheets, food diaries, and other tools can be customized to meet the individual needs of child–caregiver units so that they can work together to manage the child's diabetes and implement his or her medical regimen. It can be beneficial to monitor stress and exercise levels, in addition to diet and blood glucose testing, so that the child and caregiver gain an understanding of the need to juggle four balls when managing diabetes: food, blood glucose monitoring, exercise, and stress.

Support from her mother was critical to Jacklyn's diabetes management. This is consistent with literature indicating that family cohesion and teamwork, particularly around the child's diabetes management goals, can facilitate adherence [22]. Family meetings or finding opportunities to discuss a shared vision for diabetes management may help families find the time to plan for success and plan for monitoring the four areas for self-management (food, blood glucose monitoring, exercise, and stress). It is noteworthy that the role of the diabetes educator could be played by other health professionals such as the school nurse, the nurse on the medical team, a doctor, or a child health psychologist. Moreover, support need not always be in person or in the same setting or room. For instance, Nicholas and colleagues [13] found that participation in an online support and education program facilitated diabetes management. We believe that more research into the utility of online support is needed, as this type of support may be critical to those children and adolescents residing in rural areas where they are not close to a children's medical center. Whether it is online or in person, some of the key ingredients to adherence success are support, monitoring, and teamwork to help the child learn greater self-management.

8.2. Case study 2

Raphael is a 16-year-old male diagnosed as obese and as having T2DM related to his obesity. He is struggling with issues related to adhering to recommendations to facilitate weight loss and improve his involvement in regular physical activity, which at the current time is walking. Raphael finds walking boring and does not want any people in his neighborhood to see him walking. He reported that there was no healthy food at home and that if he ate healthy food at lunch at school, he would face teasing from his friends with whom he eats lunch. Raphael was referred for counseling by the medical team at the obesity management clinic at a local hospital. The medical team in this clinic is assisting in managing Raphael's weight management and diabetes, with consultation from a pediatric endocrinologist. In his first counseling session, Raphael stated that he felt change in his eating and exercise habits was not possible. He also admitted to having difficulty remembering to take his diabetes medication. He reported he takes his medicine about 50% of the time. His grades at school are in the "B" range, and he said he got along well with his mother, a single parent. He never sees his father and is an only child. After coming home from school, he snacks and plays video games. He has a great love of electronics, and some day he would like to have a job developing video games.

Raphael was slow to warm up to interacting with his counselor. He stated, "I'm fine and don't need to be here." The counselor attempted to establish common ground with Raphael and confirm his need to attend some counseling to learn about ways to better manage his health issues. His counselor was a male and tried to engage Raphael in conversations about video games. This was an activity Raphael liked, so he told his counselor about some games he enjoyed. Raphael particularly enjoyed games where he played against other teenagers online. After this discussion, Raphael's counselor asked if he could provide Raphael with education about diabetes management, and Raphael reluctantly agreed to discuss this.

The counselor, who was well versed in pediatric health issues, provided Raphael with information about the long-term and short-term health risks associated with his weight and diabetes. He provided Raphael with pamphlets that had information about diabetes management. He and Raphael reviewed information about diabetes from the American Diabetes Association on the counselor's laptop computer. Raphael showed surprise when learning the severity of some of the medical complications associated with T2DM. He reported, "I didn't think it was that important to take my pills or to count my carbs."

After several sessions, Raphael and his counselor agreed to a plan to improve his adherence to taking his medications and improving his diet. They involved his mother in a session, and with her assistance, they talked about having more vegetables and fruits in the refrigerator and about buying less of the high-fat, high-carbohydrate snacks that Raphael was used to consuming while he played video games in the kitchen after school. They agreed to have fruits and vegetables with light dressing available for snacks, and Raphael agreed to play video games in his room after he had his afterschool snack and tested his blood sugar. This would make it more difficult to access snacks without thinking about getting up and leaving the games in which he was involved.

Raphael also agreed to keep a calendar to monitor taking his medication every day. He agreed to take his medication in the morning, with his mother observing his actions. After taking the medication, his mother would record successful administration of the medication on the calendar. This was to occur for 1 month, and if Raphael established a regular routine for taking his medication, then he and his mother would talk about gradually turning over responsibility for taking his medication to Raphael.

A similar plan was developed for helping Raphael to begin to count his carbohydrate intake and record his snacks using a food diary. Both Raphael and his mother recorded what he ate during the day and in the evenings. His mother took notes and recorded what Raphael ate daily, and they talked about his calorie intake, how many carbohydrates he had eaten, and how often he had tested his blood sugar. Raphael was to record his blood sugar levels after school, but he was having difficulty doing this, so his mother assisted with recording this, in the hopes that after some time with this added support, Raphael would be able to record results of his daily blood glucose testing and his diet more independently. Raphael seemed to enjoy the help from his mother and her support. He did not wish to be responsible for monitoring on his own, so this shared management approach was successful. His counselor invited his mother to every third counseling session, and they had weekly phone sessions so that the counselor could support Raphael's mother's involvement in this shared management approach. Raphael's counselor contacted the nurse on his medical team and his mother also reported on their progress to the medical team. After communicating, it was agreed that referral to a nutrition expert at the hospital was necessary to gain further information and to educate Raphael and his mother further regarding weight loss and diet.

Progress was very slow in terms of improving physical activity. Raphael did not want to participate in gym class—he usually sat on the sidelines. The reason for this is he did not want to be made fun of by peers for being overweight and unable to play games well. For similar reasons, fear of teasing and stigma due to his weight, Raphael did not want to exercise in the neighborhood at home. In order to improve his access to a place where he could exercise, Raphael's counselor called a local training center. The counselor networked with the medical team to write an application to the training center so that Raphael could get a complimentary membership, as Raphael's mother could not afford to pay for a gym membership for her son. Raphael's mother worked with the counselor to develop an incentive for Raphael to work out. She agreed to reward Raphael for weekly physical activity by providing him with an allowance that he could spend on computer games. A month after joining the gym, Raphael went for a first training session. He agreed to walk on the indoor track, but not to lift weights. He was able to go to the gym once per week and was earning some extra money for video games, but progress in this area was slow and an area for continued planning and discussion in counseling sessions.

Raphael and his mother were referred to online support groups for parents and youth with diabetes after a period of time. Raphael's mother reported that she benefitted from her participation in the parent group. However, Raphael did not connect with others in his adolescent group. Therefore, the counselor contacted his medical team to see if there were other peers with which Raphael could be connected. The nurse for the team could not identify any peer support that would be a "match" for Raphael from among their current records, but the team (counselor, mother, and medical professionals) supporting Raphael all became aware of his need for peer support in coping with being overweight and having T2DM. They kept in touch through monthly telephone meetings coordinated by Raphael's counselor. Raphael continued in counseling, and his sessions were now biweekly. He enjoyed his referral to the nutrition expert and agreed to meet with her once per month.

http://dx.doi.org/10.5772/60567

In summary, Raphael showed some improvement in his diabetes management and in thinking about weight loss. Planning was in place to ensure long-term medical monitoring and support for Raphael from his mother and the medical team. This additional level of accountability was in place to improve his chances at monitoring his diabetes and weight issues. After 6 months, he was taking his medication regularly, and his snacking was healthier in nature because he was consuming more fruits and vegetables rather than potato chips and candy. He was monitoring his blood glucose levels as well. His exercise level had not greatly improved, and this was an area for continued goal setting. Eventually, it was hoped that his mother would provide less support and that Raphael would become more involved in managing his diabetes and caring for his health. This fictional case provides examples of how a counselor (and this role could also be played by other health professionals) can be an integral part of the diabetes team to help an adolescent with diabetes management. This case outlined the need for close collaboration between the parent, child, and medical team and the need for a long-term commitment to improving adherence and supporting the adolescent in order for him to learn more about his condition and become more involved in self-care. Also, this case review highlighted the importance of parent support and shared parent–child management of the diabetes regimen.

8.3. Case study 3

Jonas, a 15-year-old male with T1DM, came to his medical team because he was experiencing teasing related to needing privacy to test his blood glucose levels at school. He had requested to leave the classroom to "give myself my needle stick" to test my blood sugar. His teacher was not understanding of his need for privacy. His teacher mentioned this in front of the class, and after this incident, another boy in his class started calling him a "sissy" for his requests to "test" outside the classroom. Jonas wished to test his blood sugar levels outside the classroom so he did not feel like "everyone is 'staring at me' when I need to stick my finger with a needle to test my blood sugar."

Jonas mentioned this problem to a nurse on his diabetes management team when he came in for a regular visit with his team at a local children's hospital. The nurse recommended that Jonas have a talk with his teacher about his diabetes. Jonas replied, "Again? I have talked with him before. He doesn't listen." The nurse also had an opportunity to talk with Jonas's mother about his diabetes management at school. His mother mentioned that it was difficult for Jonas to have snacks in the classroom if his blood sugar level was low. Also, it was difficult for him to get permission to go and see the school nurse if he felt he needed her assistance if he thought his blood sugar levels were either too high or too low. After a brief conversation with the team, his nurse asked Jonas and his mother if they could talk by telephone later on the same day, after clinic had ended. The nurse for the medical team called Jonas and his mother and placed them on speaker phone so that she and Jonas's doctor could converse with Jonas and his mother about diabetes management at school.

During this conversation, both Jonas and his mother indicated that support at school for testing, snacking, and diabetes management was "below average" this year. Although support had been good in some of the previous years, it tended to change based on the classroom teacher and the changes in personnel, in terms of school nursing. The doctor brought up the need for written, special education planning as part of Jonas's school record in order to ensure that he could check his blood sugar and snack to follow his diabetes regimen. Jonas was hesitant about having a special plan, but his mother thought it would be important. The adults promised Jonas that having a special plan at school, in terms of a section 504 plan or other health impaired plan, would help Jonas, in that he would no longer need to worry about asking his teacher to test and have snacks when he needed them. After another round of discussion in the telephone conference, Jonas reluctantly agreed for his mother to approach the school staff (school principal and school nurse) about having a written health care plan for Jonas at school. His mother promised the medical team she would contact them about her progress.

Jonas's mother met with the school principal and nurse. At first, they did not wish to develop a written plan, but his mother requested a written health care plan be developed for her son's school record. She had been advised by the medical team to make sure a written health care plan, with information for handling emergency situations, was developed for the school setting. The principal and nurse agreed to this plan and a second meeting was set. This meeting included the principal, the school nurse, Jonas's mother, the nurse from Jonas's hospital-based medical care team, and his teacher. Jonas was present as well, for part of the meeting. During this meeting, a school health care plan was drafted. It included an agreement to allow Jonas to go outside the classroom to test his blood sugar level, and it required snacks to be kept in the classroom. If Jonas was experiencing a hyperglycemic or hypoglycemic episode, then a friend or classmate would walk to the nurse with him. The school nurse and his teachers, as well as the front office staff, had a special health care card with what to do if Jonas needed immediate medical attention related to his diabetes. The nurse on Jonas's medical team visited his classroom to explain his diabetes and needs for monitoring and medical management, in an effort to increase understanding and acceptance among his classmates.

In the long run, after the plan was implemented, Jonas said it was beneficial because he did not have to keep re-explaining about his diabetes to his teacher. The teacher reported increased confidence for assisting Jonas with managing his diabetes. His mother reported hearing fewer complaints from Jonas about his diabetes management at school. Written care plans can benefit children in school settings. In addition, our team believes that written care plans can help coaches and other leaders of extracurricular activities assist children with managing their diabetes and will provide important instruction about emergency planning. Written care plans should include information about eating, snacking, insulin administration, testing, and emergency planning and contacts. These plans can be a protective factor for youth with diabetes.

9. Conclusion

This chapter has presented information on areas that influence children's adherence and variables that influence children's abilities to adhere to their medical regimens. The research we have reviewed emphasizes the importance of teamwork between the child and the family

http://dx.doi.org/10.5772/60567

for establishing goals. We think that teamwork is critical, and we would like to add that the medical team is a key player on the team. When these professionals emphasize patient-centered care (with parent involvement) and goal setting, they will gain advantages in meeting children and parents "where they are" and developing specific, individualized plans to help children manage their diabetes regimen over time, thereby reducing health risks and improving quality of life and health outcomes for these children.

We have several ideas for future research to advance the field. For example, conducting more research about ways to optimize diabetes management in schools and during extracurricular after-school activities will provide information about what works best in real-world settings. Further information about "best practices" for improving adherence in children with special needs will extend the literature. Similarly, more information is needed about programs for improving diabetes management in children and adolescents with T2DM. Since many children with T2DM may be overweight, it will be important to incorporate diabetes education and awareness into weight management programs, so that youth with weight problems who develop T2DM have support for their diabetes management within the context of their weight management treatment. Perhaps researchers can utilize studies with adults with T2DM as a starting point for developing interventions to improve adherence for adolescents with T2DM since the majority of youth with T2DM will probably be in this development period.

Venditti et al. [36] discussed lifestyle coaching as an intervention to improve diabetes management. We believe that peer support from other youth with diabetes and lifestyle coaching are underexplored interventions for improving youth adherence. Peer support can occur in online or "in person" though support groups and may be an inexpensive way to provide education and support for children and adolescents with diabetes, especially during the first few years after receiving a diagnosis. Parent or caregiver support groups could work in a similar fashion to provide education and support for parents of young children who have recently been diagnosed with diabetes. Peer and parent support can also be critical when adherence becomes difficult, such as during the teenage years or after a difficult life period for youth that has been filled with significant life stressors. Understanding ways to involve peers in positive ways, to make sure that peer support has a positive and uplifting impact on emotional functioning and diabetes management, also remains important to ensuring that peer support results in positive health and emotional outcomes for youth with diabetes.

Author details

Laura Nabors*, Teminijesu John Ige, Alicia Aikens, Chris Berry, Bradley Fevrier and Patrice DeLeon

*Address all correspondence to: naborsla@ucmail.uc.edu

Health Promotion and Education Program, School of Human Services, University of Cincinnati, Cincinnati, OH, USA

References

[1] Centers for Disease Control and Prevention. Diabetes in youth. http://www.cdc.gov/diabetes/risk/age/youth.html (accessed 15 January 2015).

[2] Centers for Disease Control and Prevention. National Diabetes Statistics Report: Estimates of Diabetes and Its Burden in the United States. Atlanta, GA: U.S. Department of Health and Human Services; 2014. http://www.cdc.gov/diabetes/pubs/statsreport14/national-diabetes-report-web.pdf (accessed 15 January 2015).

[3] Botero D, Wolfsdorf JI. Diabetes mellitus in children and adolescents. Archives of Medical Research 2005;36(3);281–290. doi: 10.1016/j.arcmed.2004.12.002.

[4] National Diabetes Education Program. Overview of diabetes in children and adolescents. http://ndep.nih.gov/media/Overview-of-Diabetes-Children-508_2014.pdf (accessed 15 January 2015).

[5] American Diabetes Association. Nutritional principles and recommendations in diabetes. Diabetes Care 2004, Supplement 1, S36–S46. http://care.diabetesjournals.org/content/27/suppl_1/s36.full (accessed 15 January 2015). doi: 10.2337/diacare.27.2007.S36, Diabetes Care January 2004, 27(Suppl 1), s36.

[6] Li C, Ford ES, Zhao G, Mokdad AH. Prevalence of pre-diabetes and its association with clustering of cardiometabolic risk factors and hyperinsulinemia among U.S. adolescents: National Health and Nutrition Examination Survey 2005–2006. Diabetes Care 2009;32(2):342–347. doi: 10.2337/dc08-1128.

[7] Giannini, C., de Giorgis, T., Mohn, A., Chiarelli, F. Role of physical exercise in children and adolescents with diabetes mellitus. Journal of Pediatric Endocrinology and Metabolism 2007;20(2):173–184. doi: 10.1515/JPEM.2007.20.2.173.

[8] World Health Organization (WHO). Adherence to long-term therapies: evidence for action. In: E. Sabaté (ed.). Geneva, Switzerland: World Health Organization; 2003. ISBN 9241545992. Order no. 1150526.

[9] Amed S, Nuernberger K, McCrea P, Reimer K, Krueger H, Aydede SK, et al. Adherence to clinical practice guidelines in the management of children, youth, and young adults with type 1 diabetes: a prospective population cohort study. Journal of Pediatrics 2013;163(2):543–548. doi: http://dx.doi.org/10.1016/j.jpeds.2013.01.070.

[10] Today Study Group. A clinical trial to maintain glycemic control in youth with type 2 diabetes. New England Journal of Medicine 2012;366:2247–2256. doi: 10.1056/NEJMoa 1109333.

[11] Buckloh LM, Lochrie AS, Antal H, Milkes MA, Atilio Canas J, Hutchinson S, Wysocki T. Diabetes complications in youth: qualitative analysis of parents' perspectives of family learning and knowledge. Diabetes Care 2008;31(8):1516–1520. doi: 10.2337/dc07-2349. PMCID: PMC2494644.

[12] Marrero DG, Ard J, Delamater AM, Peragallo-Dittko V, Mayer-Davis EJ, Nwankwo R, Fisher EB. Twenty-first century behavioral medicine: a context for empowering clinicians and patients with diabetes: a consensus report. Diabetes Care 2013;36(2): 463–470. doi: 10.2337/dc12-2305.

[13] Nicholas DB, Fellner KD, Frank M, Small M, Hetherington R, Slater R, Daneman D. Evaluation of an online education and support intervention for adolescents with diabetes. Social Work in Health Care 2012; 51(9): 815–827. doi: 10.1080/00981389.2012.699507.

[14] Delamater AM, Patiño-Fernández AM, Smith KE, Bubb J. Measurement of diabetes stress in older children and adolescents with type 1 diabetes mellitus. Pediatric Diabetes 2013;14(1):50–56. doi: 10.1111/j.1399-5448.2012.00894.x.

[15] Walders-Abramson N, Venditti EM, Ievers-Landis CE, Anderson B, Geffner M, Kaplan J, Koontz MB, Saletsky R, Payan M. Relationships among stressful life events and physiological markers, treatment adherence, and psychosocial functioning among youth with type 2 diabetes. Journal of Pediatrics 2014;165(3): 504–508.e1. doi: http://dx.doi.org/10.1016/j.jpeds.2014.05.020.

[16] Hood KK, Huestis S, Maher A, Butler D, Volkening L, Laffel LMB. Depressive symptoms in children and adolescents with type 1 diabetes: association with diabetes-specific characteristics. Diabetes Care 2006;29(6):1389–1391. doi: 10.2337/dc06-0087.

[17] Kongkaew C, Jampachaisri K, Chaturongkul CA, Scholfield CN. Depression and adherence to treatment in diabetic children and adolescents: a systematic review and meta-analysis of observational studies. European Journal of Pediatrics 2014;173(2): 203–212. doi: 10.1007/s00431-013-2128-y.

[18] Herzer M, Hood KK. Anxiety symptoms in adolescents with t 1 diabetes: association with blood glucose monitoring and glycemic control. Journal of Pediatric Psychology 2010;35(4):415–425. doi: 10.1093/jpepsy/jsp063.

[19] Kovacs M, Goldston D, Obrosky DS, Bonar LK. (1997). Psychiatric disorders in youths with IDDM: rates and risk factors. Diabetes Care 1997;20(1):36–44. doi: 10.2337/diacare.20.1.36.

[20] Davison KA, Negrato CA, Cobas R, Matheus A, Tannus L, Palma CS, et al. (Brazilian Study Group, 2014). Relationship between adherence to diet, glycemic control and cardiovascular risk factors in patients with type 1 diabetes: a nationwide survey in Brazil. Nutrition Journal 2014;13(1):19. doi: 10.1186/1475-2891-13-19. http://www.nutritionj.com/content/13/1/19 (accessed 4 January 2015).

[21] Patton SR. Adherence to diet in youth with type 1 diabetes. Journal of the American Dietetic Association 2011; 111(4):550–555. doi: 10.1016/j.jada.2011.01.016.

[22] Patton SR, Dolan LM, Chen M, Powers SW. Dietary adherence and mealtime behaviors in young children with type 1 diabetes on intensive insulin therapy. Journal of

the Academy of Nutrition and Dietetics 2013;113(2):258–262. doi: 10.1016/j.jand. 2012.09.013.

[23] Quirk H, Blake H, Tennyson R, Randell TL, Glazebrook C. Physical activity interventions in children and young people with type 1 diabetes mellitus: a systematic review with meta-analysis. Diabetic Medicine 2014;31(10):1163–1173. doi: 10.1111/dme. 12531.

[24] Almeida AC, Grac⊚a-Pereira M, Engra'cia L. The influence of family support, parental coping and school support on adherence to type 1 diabetes' self-care in adolescents. In Escher A (ed.), Type 1 Diabetes. ISBN: 978-953-51-1017-0. Croatia: InTech; 2013. doi: 10.5772/53062. http://www.intechopen.com/books/type-1-diabetes/the-influence-of-family-support-parental-coping-and-school-support-on-adherence-to-type-1-diabetes-s.

[25] Lewin AB, Heidgerken AD, Geffken, GR, Williams LB, Storch EA, Gelfand KM, Silverstein JH. The relation between family factors and metabolic control: the role of diabetes adherence. Journal of Pediatric Psychology 2006;31(2):174–183. doi: 10.1093/ jpepsy/jsj004.

[26] Osborn P, Berg C, Hughes A, Pham P, Wiebe D. (2013). What mom and dad don't know can hurt you: adolescent disclosure to and secrecy from parents about type 1 diabetes. Journal of Pediatric Psychology 2013;38(2):141–150. doi: 10.1093/jpepsy/ jss102.

[27] Miller VA, Jawad AF. Relationship of youth involvement in diabetes-related decisions to treatment adherence. Journal of Clinical Psychology in Medical Settings 2014;21(2):183–189. doi: 10.1007/s10880-014-9388-1.

[28] Nabors L, Lehmkuhl H, Christos N, Andreone TL. Children with diabetes: perceptions of supports for self-management at school. Journal of School Health 2013;73(6): 216–221. doi: 10.1111/j.1746-1561.2003.tb06563.x.

[29] American Diabetes Association. Diabetes care in the school and day care setting. Diabetes Care 2012;35(Supplement 1): S76-S80. doi: 10.2337/dc12-s076.

[30] Ritholz MD, Beverly EA, Weinger K. Digging deeper: the role of qualitative research in behavioral diabetes. Current Diabetes Reports 2011;11(6):494–502. doi: 10.1007/ s11892-011-0226-7.

[31] Hood KK, Peterson CM, Rohan JM, Drotar D. Association between adherence and glycemic control in pediatric type 1 diabetes: a meta-analysis. Pediatrics 2009;124(6): e1171-e1179.doi: 10.1542/peds.2009-0207.

[32] Katz ML, Volkening LK, Butler DA, Anderson BJ, Laffel LM. Family-based psychoeducation and care ambassador intervention to improve glycemic control in youth with type 1 diabetes: a randomized trial. Pediatric Diabetes 2014;15(2):142–150. doi: 10.1111/pedi.12065.

[33] Boogerd EA, Noordam C, Verhaak CM. The Sugarsquare Study: protocol of a multicenter randomized controlled trial concerning a web-based patient portal for parents of a child with type 1 diabetes.BMC Pediatrics 2014;14(1);24. 8 pages doi: 10.1186/1471-2431-14-24. http://www.biomedcentral.com/1471-2431/14/24 (accessed 4 January 2015).

[34] Kienle GS, Meusers M, Quecke B, Hilgard D. Patient-centered diabetes care in children: an integrated, individualized, systems-oriented, and multidisciplinary approach. Global Advances in Health and Medicine 2013;2(2):12–19. doi: 10.7453/gahmj.2013.005.

[35] Miller V, Drotar D. Decision-making competence and adherence to treatment in adolescents with diabetes. Journal of Pediatric Psychology 2007;32(2):178–188. doi: 10.1093/jpepsy/jsj122.

[36] Venditti E, Wylie-Rosett J, Delahanty L, Mele L, Hoskin M, Edestein S. for the Diabetes Prevention Group. Short and long-term lifestyle coaching approaches used to address diverse participant barriers to weight loss and physical activity adherence. International Journal of Behavioral Nutritional and Physical Activity, 2014;11. (16). http://www.ijbnpa.org/content/11/1/16 (accessed 15 January 2015).

[37] Bell KJ, Barclay AW, Petocz P, Colagiuri S, Branú-Miller JC. Efficacy of carbohydrate counting in type 1 diabetes: a systematic review and meta-analysis. Lancet Diabetes and Endocrinology 2014; 2(2): 133–140. doi: http://dx.doi.org/10.1016/S2213-8587(13)70144-X (accessed 4 January 2015).

[38] Shulman RM, Daneman D. Type 1 diabetes mellitus in childhood. Medicine 2010, 38(12), 679–685. doi: 10.1016/j.mpmed.2010.09.001.